The Heroics
of Falling Apart

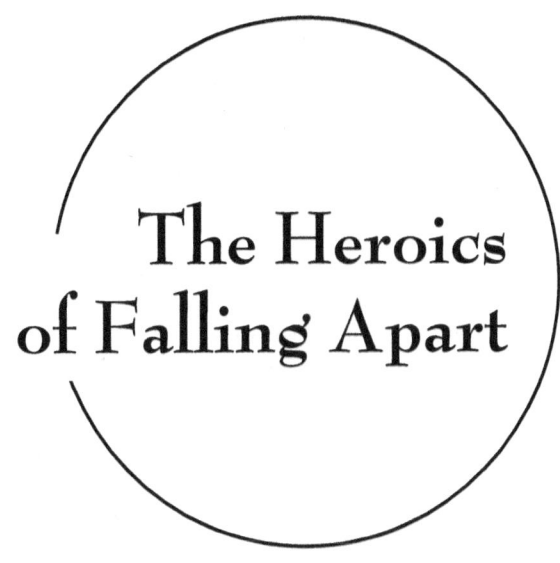

The Heroics
of Falling Apart

One Couple's Breast Cancer Journey

Judy Gordon and Dan Gordon

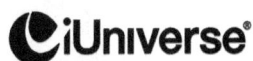

The Heroics of Falling Apart
One Couple's Breast Cancer Journey

iUniverse books may be ordered through booksellers or by contacting:

iUniverse
1663 Liberty Drive
Bloomington, IN 47403
www.iuniverse.com
844-349-9409

Because of the dynamic nature of the Internet, any web addresses or links contained in this book may have changed since publication and may no longer be valid. The views expressed in this work are solely those of the author and do not necessarily reflect the views of the publisher, and the publisher hereby disclaims any responsibility for them.

Any people depicted in stock imagery provided by Getty Images are models, and such images are being used for illustrative purposes only.
Certain stock imagery © Getty Images.

ISBN: 978-0-5954-1911-1 (sc)
ISBN: 978-0-5958-6258-0 (e)

Print information available on the last page.

iUniverse rev. date: 07/23/2020

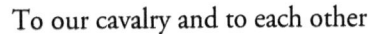

To our cavalry and to each other

Contents

Acknowledgments

Writing a book about our experience with cancer was the last thing on our minds as we approached the final treatment stage some eighteen months after Judy's diagnosis. Our lives had been invaded and taken over by that unwelcome guest, and all we were interested in was getting to the point where we no longer had to frame our lives around a disease. Yet as time went on, more and more people encouraged Judy to write and share these memoirs. In some way, they sensed that the experience of revisiting the journey would prove therapeutic, thought-provoking, revealing, and often hilarious. Judy agreed to take on the endeavor, and for all those who planted and then watered that seed, we are forever grateful.

It was Scotty Dupree who, upon hearing Judy's plans for a book, suggested that Dan contribute to the effort. Scotty felt that Judy and Dan writing about the experience together would have great personal benefits for each of us. She was right. Dan had gone through the entire cancer journey in a state of self-imposed stoicism, something he needed to do to help both of us get through it. Writing about it so comprehensively gave him the opportunity to finally experience the journey emotionally. Judy, who had kept a journal throughout the experience, found there were still many ideas and thoughts that needed to be expressed and revisited from a healthier perspective.

Writing this together allowed us—and forced us—to sift through and find the essence of the experience in its entirety as well as its individual moments along the way. We discovered that what the other was going through was not always evident while it was going on, and we learned that we could remember the exact same event in very different ways. Even more important, revisiting that era in our lives allowed us to rediscover each other and renew our relationship. Making this memoir a joint project felt like the final step in completing our cancer journey, and we are thankful we were talked into it.

We thank our friend Scott Sawyer, conveniently a writer and editor himself, who volunteered to be our first reader. He eagerly and thoughtfully went through our initial draft, positively critiquing and directing our effort into something more than we had imagined it could be.

Another friend, Annie Zook, was not only a constant and creative support during the worst of the journey, but she also helped us capture some of the important visuals, including the cover photos.

They say it takes a village to raise a child. But it also takes a village to support people through this sort of life-changing event; and sometimes, as we learned, that village comes in the guise of cavalry. We are so grateful for ours—our children and their families, Judy's sisters, our friends, and all the people we met along the way. You inspire us.

Introduction

JUDY

My husband, Dan, and I have been a partnership for almost forty years now, and we've always used "we" when we talk about our shared life. The cancer journey did not divide that partnership. Dan was present for all procedures and appointments. He always listened; he advised when asked; and he took charge when needed. He loved and supported me unconditionally. "Nothing's too scary if we can talk about it; nothing's too scary if we can laugh about it," he'd say. We relied on our partnership and took comfort in each other. We shared this journey together, so it only made sense that we'd also share in the writing of this memoir.

It's been three years since my diagnosis, and I like to think I am feeling 100 percent my old self. But that's not quite accurate. I will never be my old self again because I emerged from the journey a different person. That's only natural—any person going through the cancer experience should expect to be altered by it.

I wouldn't say I came out of the experience as a *warrior*, though that is a word that many cancer patients and survivors use to describe themselves. I didn't see cancer as something to wage a battle against. Instead, I chose a less common, less popular way to cope with the diagnosis and treatment. Maybe I'm wrong: perhaps the road I chose to take is typical, but if it is, that way isn't celebrated much, probably because it's not very glamorous or heroic. In truth, the road I took was probably far too messy for anyone who witnessed my journey to blithely say, "Yeah, that's the way I want to do it."

On the other hand, *surrender* might also be too strong a word to describe my reaction to cancer. Perhaps *going with the flow* is a more accurate description, albeit a somewhat abstract concept. It's fitting, because there is a lot of abstraction in one's own dealing with cancer. It's an unknown journey. Cancer affects all aspects of a person's life in unpredictable and unique ways.

Perhaps the best spin to put on my journey was that I simply did it my way. And as it turned out, that was the only way I could have done it if I wanted to survive. And I did survive, but to do that, I had to fall apart. People who inquire about my experience receive my candid reply: I literally fell apart. I want to be authentic in my replies, just as I had been authentic in letting my emotions rule me at times while I went through the experience.

I remember most of the experience vividly, because I kept a journal of my cancer journey for over a year. In the following chapters, I've included bits and pieces of that recollection. But these memories became so much richer after I added my reflections on what the journey has meant to me.

DAN

I am not an emotional person. In fact, displays of emotion, whether verbal or physical, embarrass me. I don't know how to respond to them. I do react, but I wonder as I'm doing so whether I reacted appropriately. What's worse for me than being present during someone else's emotional display are those rare occasions when my own well-repressed emotion decides it needs to see the light of day. When this happens, the emotion usually sneaks out when I am alone, making it easier to deal with. But when the release finally comes, the emotion is pretty determined to be expressed.

Containing my feelings is usually my primary instinct, but once in a while an emotion manifests itself in me in the form of watery eyes or a quivering voice. Then, only after I know that I have safely confined the emotion once again I can objectively ask myself, "What the hell brought that on?"

My emotional triggers usually include a scene in a movie or lyrics in a song. Never anything real. Not something or someone in my presence. Real life doesn't move me. Somewhere, somehow, I learned to numb my emotions, to insulate all but my intellectual faculties. Life, with all its emotional vagaries, is to be endured and understood logically, but not felt. I believed that was an OK, acceptable way to live. But it also made me probably the worst person to be put in the role of caregiver—for anyone, let alone my wife and best friend of almost forty years. So naturally, given the universe's fondness for irony, that is exactly where I found myself when Judy was diagnosed with breast cancer.

My unsuitability for a part, however, has never stopped me from accepting whatever role life has presented me. Whenever I am faced with doing something I don't think I want to do or wouldn't be very good at, a sense of responsibility and adventure takes precedent. I never imagined myself as a parent, but I liked the things that led to becoming one, so when the time came I gladly took on that role. I never had a strong affinity for work, but given my love for Judy and the family that came of that love, I gladly, and somewhat successfully, played my part as a breadwinner. And when the word came that Judy was looking at a rough time ahead, both physically and emotionally, I geared up to be the support system she would need.

But I wasn't emotionally involved in the experience until much later. Too much happened too quickly once the diagnosis was made. The cancer instantly impacted all aspects of our life. As was her nature and under the circumstances, Judy gave free rein to her emotions. I, however, held mine in check. That can be seen as a good thing. My being strong and grounded for both of us would help us through the difficult times. It may even have been the best way for me to be. But despite my outward demeanor, the emotions were still there, more varied and intense than I ever could have guessed at the time. It was only when I began writing my part of these memoirs and reading Judy's excerpts that I realized the extent and depth of the emotions involved, and I felt them as well.

That doesn't mean I breezed through Judy's experience fulfilling my caregiver responsibilities with the detached air of a professional. The emotional upheaval I denied did surface, but usually in other forms. Often it came out as anger—anger randomly directed at my work, other drivers, a disappointing movie, or whoever or whatever crossed my path when I needed to vent. And I needed to vent more often than I'm comfortable admitting. I also experienced a fair amount of self-pity. At times I martyred myself to the caregiver role, using it as an excuse not to do something for myself. On other occasions the self-pity took the form of worry—but not *the* worry. It was more a fretting over little things, such as the logistics of arranging to meet someone, having all the right stuff for dinner, or needing to take more time off from work for yet another doctor's appointment.

The big worry, however, made its way to the surface a couple times. Like the night Judy told me that if she ever had to go through cancer treatment again, she wouldn't. That was a big-worry moment for me that lingered because after she said it she went up to bed, leaving me with a long evening to ponder all that those few words meant. I would have preferred that she exit the scene with a more positive and hopeful remark. Something that would not only inspire but also fill me with a sense of pride and make me want to puff up and shout to the world, "That's my woman. So brave. So strong. An inspiration to us all." Instead I heard complete resignation in her words. Surrender. Implied in that surrender was the possibility of losing her, a reality I refused to consider throughout the journey. So instead of addressing that underlying fear, I allowed myself to be disappointed. Disappointed that she wasn't handling things in the way that I would have liked her to. Disappointed that she wasn't fighting harder.

But fighting seemed to be *the* problem for Judy. The conventional wisdom about cancer is that a person needs to fight it. Whether it's a magazine article about some cancer-stricken celebrity or somebody's obituary notice, the emphasis always lies on heroically battling against the disease. The individual's ordeal is elevated to something that's noble and purposeful, with cancer personified as the evil enemy. That imagery is functional: if the patient buys into it, there is motivation and distraction to help the person get through the worst. But while inspiring images of battles bravely fought may conjure uplifting thoughts to some, Judy is a pacifist at heart. To her, battles only suggest casualties. Down deep she probably felt that if she didn't go to war with cancer, even metaphorically, then she would avoid being a casualty. Under different circumstances I might have viewed that as heroic in its own right. Unfortunately, flashing the peace sign at the juggernaut bursting through her door spared Judy none of the consequences. No terms were offered simply because Judy refused to fight back. Cancer came and attacked her full force, and I witnessed her wither before it. I thought she needed to do something more; falling apart did not seem enough of a response.

The overlooked part of our—and I suspect other people's—cancer experience was that it forced not just Judy as the cancer victim but also me as the caregiver to reevaluate and redefine who we thought we were. We had to make some fundamental adjustments. Yes, I wanted Judy to battle her cancer, but in the immediacy and reality of the moment, I had to defer to her and then actively support her way of dealing with it. In retrospect, it is easy to see that doing so was the *only* way.

JUDY

While I was self-absorbed with my treatment, side effects, and emotions, Dan was not only managing his own demons but mine as well. His expression of that experience in these memoirs has given me an even deeper appreciation of what he went through and how he viewed what was happening to me. There is a richness in his pages that makes my heart almost burst. I am grateful to have such a loving partner who is committed to not only working through difficult situations but also willing to speak the truth about them. I know other men will see themselves in his candid descriptions and will gain understanding and confidence as they uncover their own commitments and strategies in dealing with such an insidious disease or other life-threatening experience.

A long time ago, in 1974 to be exact, Dan and I became parents for the first time. Unlike previous generations, we were part of a culture that sought to bring a woman and a man together to experience their child's birth. We took one of the earliest Lamaze classes at our hospital in Springfield, Illinois. Excited about preparing for that special moment, we took our learning very seriously. We were in the forefront of a movement that would forever banish the isolation of dads and other partners from the labor and delivery room. We were thrilled to lean on each other in such a new adventure.

Like those early days when men and women first shared the experience of childbirth together, today men and women share the experience of cancer and other health problems. But today, there is no equivalent to the Lamaze class for couples experiencing such an illness together. So couples need to hear from others who have traveled and suffered the same path. Although our journey was unwelcome, it also held its own knowledge and gifts. Our hope is that we can share the knowledge we gained with other couples, and that our tale will support them as they walk a similar road and share in their unique foray together. Such a partnership will help make the decisions easier to make, the bad days better, and the seemingly impossible, possible.

January 2007

1

Race for the Cure 2003: Hey, Gang, Let's Pick Up the Pace

JUDY

After fifteen years of normal results from mammograms, it certainly wasn't on my radar screen to be worried about breast cancer. I was only fifty-five. Healthy. And I was diligent about checkups, not just my mammogram. I had an annual pap smear, I went to the dentist twice a year, I went to the eye doctor twice a year, and I had my cholesterol tested annually. I was on medication for high cholesterol and watched what I ate. Yes, I was always ten pounds heavier than I would like to be, but it wasn't from eating unhealthy foods—it was just from eating portions that were bigger than I needed. I did a variety of exercise—walking, yoga, folk dancing, swimming—and not just for the health or weight-loss benefits. I did them because I really enjoyed them.

Not only was I healthy in October 2003, but I was also very happy. My life was sweet—idyllic almost—and practically stress-free. I have always had an optimistic outlook. I had no reason not to. My riches were abundant: a happy marriage of thirty-three years, two grown sons on their own yet still happily connected to us, two fun and healthy grandchildren to make life even sweeter, a comfortable home, and many good and close friends. I had a lot to appreciate, and I did appreciate it all.

And then, on top of being healthy and happy, I was also busy, and meaningfully so. In my work with nonprofit organizations, I addressed many of life's more challenging issues and worked with countless incredible and dedicated individuals. I was content with my internal and external world.

In my leisure time I chose my causes intuitively. A storyteller for a number of years, I volunteered to enrich the classroom experience of sixth, seventh, and eighth graders once a month. Through the presentation of folk tales, I brought the students a variety of educational and entertaining messages.

Another cause I made time for, and had for a number of years, was breast cancer research. I participated in an annual fundraising event sponsored by the Susan G. Komen Breast Cancer Foundation. That year I walked in the Race for the Cure event in our hometown of Denver with my daughter-in-law, Jen, and six-month-old grandson, Spencer. In previous years I had arranged to walk with a friend, or else I just showed up on my own and let fate determine who I walked with. That year I chose to take the opportunity to make it a family day. As Jen and I walked, and after talking about a hundred other things, she asked me if I actually knew anyone who had breast cancer. I told her about my friends Gina and Cathlin, both survivors for several years at that time. I appreciated the opportunity to think of them and to give Jen a more personal connection to the purpose of our walk. As we discussed Gina and Cathlin, I never suspected that within two weeks I would be adding my name to that list.

DAN

To the best of my recollection, Judy has participated in the Race for the Cure for as long as it's been going on. Every October. I think she went even before she knew anyone close who had breast cancer. She simply felt it was a good cause to support and the right thing to do, even if there were no personal ties. I found nothing unusual in that. People, instinctively, will involve themselves with something and then, partially out of habit and partially out of intuition, stick with it. Creating routines and traditions for ourselves is part of life, so I never read anything into her participation. She was a woman, she had breasts, and she was healthy. For me, that was reason enough to lend her support to an organization seeking a cure for a disease that impacted so many healthy women like her.

In the years when we lived in a downtown Denver loft, I dropped Judy off near the starting line on my way to work. When we moved to a neighborhood just outside of downtown, our home was close enough to the starting line that Judy walked there herself. That year, 2003, Judy walked the event with our daughter-in-law, Jen, and our grandson, Spencer. They participated in the women-only phase of the event, with Spencer getting in by virtue of being only six-months-old and in a stroller. While the women and children walked, our younger son Alex and I intended to wait for them at the house, after which we would meet our other son, Darren, and then all go out to breakfast. It was too early for Alex and me to settle in front of a football game, so I suggested we walk a couple of blocks to where we could watch the participants. We could find Judy and Jen and Spencer, wave, and maybe even take their picture as they went past. It sounded like a reasonable plan until we arrived and saw just how overwhelming a swarm of fifty thousand people is. There was no way we were going to pick them out.

It was an amazing sight. From our vantage point we could view the first several blocks of the race, and that expanse was filled with endless waves of women dressed in race-day T-shirts—white for supporters, pink for survivors. It was as if some daring and twisted filmmaker remade *The Sorcerer's Apprentice* in the context of a Good & Plenty commercial. The pavement was obscured. Thousands of marching pink and white figures made their way up the hill, past where Alex and I watched in awe. Judy had told me about the previous years' turnouts, and I had read the numbers in the newspaper, but until I actually witnessed the event first-hand, I couldn't really comprehend or visualize it.

I commented to Alex about the sight in front of us, wondering what other causes might stand to benefit from such support. There were other diseases out there that were equally deserving of being the focus of public attention. Other social issues as well, including some that almost everyone could agree need to be addressed. But no other cause seemed to garner this kind of turnout, and I had to wonder why. I guess part of it had to do with sheer numbers. If one in every eight American women gets breast cancer, then almost everyone in the United States knows at least one person who has had it. But I sensed there was more to it than that. Other issues impact those kinds of numbers. I'm sure those suffering from heart disease or who are victims of crime are just as numerous. Yet no other cause inspires a response comparable to what Alex and I witnessed that day. If I were to understand the kind of turnout breast cancer generates, I would have to move out of the realm of facts and numbers and into the fuzzier world of amateur analysis. I liked the fuzzier world, where I could always find a way to explain the inexplicable, and always end up satisfied that I got an answer. Once started, the analysis quickly produced an explanation for the spectacle we were watching. The overwhelming turnout for the Race for the Cure must have had something to do with our culture's fascination with the female breast. That fascination, coupled with the proclamation of cancer as the bogeyman laureate of our age, made the massive number of race participants before me understandable. The bogeyman was attacking a cultural icon—a totally unacceptable scenario. It simply had to be stopped.

Intellectually, that hastily derived conclusion sufficed for the moment. But deep down, I could not buy into it. It wasn't the focus on the female breast that bothered me: I was sufficiently fascinated in that regard. What I couldn't buy into was cancer as the official and innate bogeyman. To me, cancer was just one of many difficulties in life, one that may or may not personally impact me. It was no worse than alcoholism, car accidents, poverty, Alzheimer's, depression, or heart disease. Cancer was something to be reckoned with when it happened, but to set out to defeat it ascribed to it a determinant, intentional quality that it simply did not possess. It wasn't the devil collecting souls. It wasn't a terrorist trying to undermine our way of life. Cancer was a disease. Just one of the countless occurrences that may alter or even end our lives. Getting rid of cancer would not make any of us immortal. There would always be something else. And if the something elses were eradicated, then some new something elses would show up. We were not going to achieve immortality—at least not in this lifetime. So rather than put all that energy into defeating cancer, it made more sense to me to find ways to positively enrich life. However, even though that is the way I felt, and even though I went so far as to share those thoughts with Alex, I wasn't about to spend even a moment trying to sway anyone else to my way of thinking. Not in that Race for the Cure crowd. The anti-abortionists who stood in the middle of the street, defiantly preaching to the oncoming waves of pink and white their message that abortions cause breast cancer, were an object lesson in how not to display common sense and tact. My beliefs were not burning a hole in my brain, needing to get out and save the world, blinding me to the needs and hopes and intimacies of the strong. And I wasn't even going to try to sway Judy to my way of thinking. She's a bright woman who happens to occasionally view things differently than I do. That day she wanted to show her solidarity with everyone impacted by breast cancer. I was preoccupied with wanting the Broncos to defeat whomever it was they were playing that afternoon. It's an awareness of those kinds of contrasting perspectives that lead me to the laissez-"do-your-own-thing"-faire philosophy I tend to live by.

JUDY

Despite all the good karma and good health that I believed served as my shield, my annual mammogram in October 2003 indicated abnormalities. Abnormalities. The word threw me back in time.

More than twenty-five years earlier, I had experienced breast lumps—lumps that I detected myself. This was long before I was going for annual mammograms; long before there were breast centers at most hospitals. I knew that doing breast self-exams was a good preventative measure, but the amount and scope of public information about breast cancer that existed then wasn't nearly what it is today. With the first lump, a visit to my OB/GYN led immediately to an outpatient biopsy. I felt pretty confident that having found a lump and doing something about it right away would lead to a good conclusion. Since I am always anxious about medical issues, I imagine I was difficult to live with until the pathology came back negative. When I detected a second lump a few years later, it concerned me, but I sensed that it was probably similar to the first lump, and that proved to be the case. Both lumps were deemed part of a fibro-cystic condition, common to many women. Fortunately, what was a minor scare turned out to be benign.

I had not worried about my breast health since then, but that lack of worry did not make me less diligent. I did self-exams every month. In fact, a wonderful gadget reminded me to do so. Our health insurance provider sent out self-exam kits that included an electronic device that counted the days between periods and flashed red when it was the optimal time for a breast exam. I replaced the batteries in that device for many years, and it always stayed visible on our bathroom counter. I felt righteous and protected with that gadget. But in October 2003 my self-exam did not detect the abnormalities that the mammogram found.

When the clinic notified me to come back for additional views, I didn't get the sense that anything was worrisome. Sometimes technology is fussy, and a second view is needed to set the record straight. I was confident it would, and I don't remember worrying very much about the retake. I'm not sure I even told Dan about it. Fall is always a busy time for me, between work and volunteer activities, so I was pleasantly engaged and preoccupied in the ten to fourteen days between the phone call to schedule a second mammogram and the retake itself.

The retake on October 21 was actually an ultrasound. This was all new technology to me, and I had no idea the machine was powerful enough to detect cancer. Yet immediately upon seeing the picture, the breast center educator delivered exactly that news to me, and in such a way that I sensed she did not feel she was premature in doing so. The ultrasound showed a lump the size of a small pea on my left breast, fairly deep in the center toward my breast bone. It was not something I had felt in my self-exams, and it turned out to be something that was not palpable by the doctors. Its irregular edge and slight star-like webbing gave the medical professionals enough information, even before a biopsy, to suggest cancer. The left breast also showed calcifications that could be precancerous. The right breast had calcifications also, but they disappeared on further views.

I instantly felt vulnerable, shaken to my core. I had come in for a retake, and now a whole new scenario confronted me. Suddenly, something was wrong with me. What had happened? How could they tell so much from a picture? Why had I not brought Dan along with me to handle this news? How was I going to tell him? I wanted to run away from the information, and there was no holding back the tears.

But I couldn't run away or stay in tears for very long. The staff at the breast center wouldn't let me leave until they talked to me about my next step. In fact, they scheduled a core biopsy for the very next day. I tried to negotiate a delay, saying I was already busy that day. (Couldn't I stay in denial a bit longer?) But the breast center staff insisted that I have the procedure immediately. When I went to bed that night, I began to sense the surreal. I wrote in my first journal entry, *If I could just stay in this evening, the unknown would stay unknown.*

The next day found me back at the breast center, but not alone. Dan came with me, and maybe having someone else there kept me from focusing so much on the fear. As the technician explained the procedure to both of us, and Dan saw the pictures that had already been taken, I was surprised at how relaxed I was. My blood pressure was 120/65 before the procedure and 115/65 after. I gave thanks to yoga for the relaxation skills and the ability to hold a position for a length of time. Both skills came in handy over the subsequent months.

During the biopsy my senses focused in on the details of my surroundings. I hadn't had any medical procedure for more than twenty-five years and was pleasantly surprised at how the medical community was now incorporating some non-medical touches to improve the experience. They gave me a warm bathrobe to wear. Music played in a calm, soothing room. Someone actually held my hand and asked me how I was doing, giving me her full attention and a distraction to focus on.

But the pleasantness of the experience did not alter the outcome. The next morning we received the results: "ductal invasive carcinoma." The unknown had become known, and we were stunned.

DAN

Not too many days after the Race for the Cure, I was in the kitchen watching Judy come out of the garage and walk across the yard. I could see that something was wrong. By default, Judy is always up, always smiling. In the absence of intervening negative forces, Judy is hardwired to be positive and upbeat. So when I saw Judy with a furrowed brow, almost a scowl, I knew something had happened. And since she was coming from the garage, I naturally assumed it was car related. A ticket. Or an accident.

It wasn't the car. She had just returned from having her mammogram redone. I don't recall if she even told me she was going to have a retake. If she had, the retake was being done with such routine matter-of-factness that I attached no apprehension to it. The first mammogram was merely unacceptable, which was not an unusual occurrence, often indicating technical problems. Whenever a repeat is taken, however, someone reads the results right away. Judy's technician read them and told her to come back the next day for a biopsy. There was something suspicious there. The reader had even gone so far as to use the cancer word.

The furrowed brow and the scowl quickly dissolved into fear and tears. Long-time, shadowy, worst-case scenarios began to solidify, even though we knew nothing for sure. The only thing certain was that we were put into a state of limbo and would remain there for another two days, until the biopsy was done and the verdict rendered. In the meantime, diversion was the best way to cope. Fortunately, I had the following day off, so Judy would not have to wait it out alone. We would find ways to occupy our time and our minds, instead of borrowing on the turmoil of what might be coming, but also what might not.

I changed my plans for the evening, and we abandoned the day's menu plan, opting to go to a Japanese restaurant for dinner, one of our comfort spots. Television sets scattered throughout the restaurant broadcast the baseball playoffs. Either they were too strategically placed to be ignored, or we looked to them to occupy ourselves in the most vapid way we could until the food arrived. The rest of that night and the next day followed that same pattern of finding something to do, something else to think about until it was time to return to the breast center late that afternoon.

The breast center waiting room was diverting enough. I found two seats together while Judy checked in with someone she was familiar with, a too-jolly woman who always used the same tired joke about how "we're going to pick on you today." Under the circumstances, it was barely amusing the first time I heard it, and by the third time it escalated to very annoying. "Somebody should clue her in," I thought, but I understood it was the circumstances of my being there that left me so intolerant. Another time, another day, her repetitious repartee might be just what the doctor ordered. And when I looked around at the other waiting women, I saw that no one else was bothered. No one else seemed to even notice. They were all there for an annual, routine checkup, just as Judy had been a dozen days before. No one looked concerned that a checkup might lead to something less routine.

Judy and I were called into a room where someone informed us about the procedure Judy would have to undergo. Then I was shown the suspicious pictures taken the day before. I only saw white, ghostly smears against a black background. It could have been anything: Judy's breast captured by the ultrasound the day before or swirls of subatomic particles photographed with an electron microscope. Nothing registered; nothing was memorable; nothing was identifiable. Then I was told what the various shadows and shapes indicated, but I could not buy into the words. We were still in the investigative process, and until the professionals informed us of something more tangible than "suspicious," there was nothing for me to take seriously, other than Judy's worry.

When Judy was led away to do the biopsy, I was left in the empty room with endless pamphlets and a couple of videos about breast cancer, all as forgettable as they were uninviting. Instead of sampling the materials, I allowed myself to wonder if Judy had some intuitive sense that this time her fears were grounded. She seemed too worried, almost fatalistic. It was not like her to borrow trouble. She certainly had no tolerance for me when I did. And while she seemed relaxed when she returned to the room a short time later, it was an uneasy relaxed. A doctor sat down with us. He did not give us any indication of where we were headed but only assured us we would be contacted with the results in the morning. We resided in another night of limbo. Reason enough to not be relaxed.

I got the call at work late the next morning. Judy was crying but I could make out, "I've got it." I quickly arranged to leave work, and I walked into the house fifteen minutes later. I found her upstairs in the bedroom, still crying. I held her, not knowing what to say, but repeatedly assuring her that everything would turn out OK. What else was there to say or to believe? The crying subsided after a while, and she told me I shouldn't have left work, that we could have talked about the situation later. "I can always go back and finish up," I said, "but you shouldn't have to be alone right now."

I didn't know then, at least in a conscious, rational way, how much that aloneness theme would run through this whole experience. But instinctively I must have known. Reassuring her that we were in this together just popped out in that moment, possibly a product of our past experiences with cancer, but more likely it was simply a product of our history together. We had always done things together. Whatever brought my words to the surface, I understood that reaffirming the "together" concept was the first, and most important, thing to do.

But something else was happening to me. Something detached, something selfish. In that same instant, with Judy in my arms sobbing in fear and despair, I sensed something that can only be described as excitement. It did not cross my mind at the time that there was anything life threatening in Judy's diagnosis, so I was not dealing with the idea of possibly losing her. Without that concern in the picture, I was able first to realize, and then admit, that I was excited by what was happening. Not a joyful-in-the-moment excitement, but an anticipatory one. Whatever happened next would be new territory for us. Newness generates excitement. What would it be like? How would we handle it? Were permanent, life-altering changes coming, and if so, what would they be? Change was the key concept at work here. Big changes were coming—short-term ones for sure, and possibly some ongoing ones as well. Either way, for the foreseeable future, our lives were not going to be the same. A different framework would define our lives; our perceptions would be filtered through a different lens. For me, at least, it was not unlike finding out Judy was pregnant for the first time. Or when I convinced her to sell our Denver home of twenty years and move into a downtown loft. Big changes were coming. What lay ahead was unknown, but as much as anything else I was feeling, I was eager to see how everything would play out.

Naturally, that sense of selfish excitement triggered some guilt. What must be wrong with me that I could have such thoughts, so incongruous to the seriousness of the situation and so insensitive to how Judy would be impacted by the disease? But the guilt could not unseat my excitement. The unexpected feeling had quickly and firmly settled in me in total disregard of the circumstances; a rude guest not aware it was an inappropriate time to come calling. That I would keep that sense of excitement under wraps was certain. But, in retrospect, I have to wonder how helpful it was to me in the coming months that I could, in quiet moments alone, step back and detach myself from the everyday details of being a caregiver and allow myself to see things from the perspective of a sweeping life change. Exciting? For sure. Necessary? Very likely.

2

Dealing with the Old Fears and Digesting the News

JUDY

Although I was fifty-five at the time of my diagnosis, I had been worried about cancer for a very long time. Yet I cannot remember how that worry took root. In my early years, none of my relatives had cancer, but I did have one elementary-age friend who died from leukemia. That was very frightening to many of us, her peers. And it may have led to the one childhood experience that really sticks out to me, an incident in which I was completely overtaken by my fear of cancer.

When I was eleven or twelve, I was hanging out with friends at the shopping center (pre-mall days) and felt an irritation on the inside of my cheek. In my memory, it seems that I quickly thought the worst about what the irritation could be—cancer—and actually walked into a dentist's office at the shopping center (not my regular dentist) to ask for a "look-see." It's unlikely that the dentist accommodated me, and I don't remember the resolution of the incident. But it is my earliest memory of fearing cancer. Over the years I have called myself a hypochondriac, but really I didn't have the traditional symptoms of that syndrome—I worried only about getting cancer.

Later I had more concrete reasons to fear the disease. A combination of breast, colon, and liver cancer took my maternal grandmother when she was seventy-five; I was twenty-seven when it happened. My father died of lung cancer when he was fifty-four; I was thirty then, and pregnant with our second child. When my mother was seventy-three, she died from ovarian cancer; I was forty-nine. Immediately following my mother's death, a younger friend of mine was diagnosed with breast cancer, and ever since then I have been touched by a number of other people with cancer.

My cancer connection continued right up to the day before my diagnosis. On that day I had attended a conference on general nonprofit issues, during which I attended two workshops that included presentations about a local breast cancer awareness organization, Day of Caring. I had even picked up some breast cancer resource materials, not because I had a specific need for them but because I am a nonprofit professional and am interested in how nonprofits communicate their programs. Perhaps I also thought I would share the info with others. So what was the likelihood that out of twenty possible workshops I would have selected two workshops that put the breast cancer topic in front of me? I believe in synchronicity, but in hindsight, my actions were also prescient.

So when I received my own diagnosis, I was overwhelmed yet not unprepared; I had both familiarity and knowledge. "At least," I thought to myself, "I have a cancer with a greater likelihood of remission or cure than my parents' cancers." Lung cancer in 1979 was always terminal; ovarian cancer in 1997 was often terminal; breast cancer in 2003 had a much lower fatality rate.

While familiarity, knowledge, or rationalizations were useful at times, they were of little help in communicating my upsetting news to my loved ones. Informing my three sisters of my diagnosis was going to be the most difficult, in light of our parents' deaths from cancer. I am the oldest sister, and it almost felt as though my cancer was a preview of what their own futures would hold. Fortunately, testing revealed that my breast cancer and my mother's ovarian cancer do not have genetic links; just because my mother and I got ill did not mean my sisters would. But a third cancer diagnosis in the immediate family was painful—and a bit ominous.

Still, because we four sisters communicate well, I didn't hesitate for a second to share my news with the others. I'm the sole sister who left our hometown of Chicago; the other three all live in that area. I called each sister in succession—Bonnie, Laurie, and Debbie. None of them were home. My news would have to wait for their return calls, although I'm sure my message on their answering machines conveyed that I was calling about a serious matter.

When Bonnie returned the call, she was driving. Though Bonnie is my youngest sister, eleven years my junior, she is the one I have remained closest to over the years. She leads a busy life, including being the mother of two young daughters. We often talk when she is driving. This time she needed to pull over to the side of the road to digest what I was saying. And her tears flowed freely. Her best friend had lost a sister to cancer not too long before, and I'm sure that recent experience had made Bonnie highly sensitive to any similar situation in her own context.

Laurie is third in the birth order. She is a nurse, so after her initial response of shock and then her expression of love and concern for my well-being, the conversation turned to the details of the diagnosis. Because of her experience in the medical field, it was no surprise that she wanted to know the details of my condition. That was nicely diverting. Discussing the situation objectively helped me get more comfortable with the new language we were having to learn.

Debbie is closest to me in age and is the sister who has carved out the most unique and unconventional way in the world. She is a single parent of a grown daughter and has always been entrepreneurial in her work. She happens to be squeamish when it comes to medical talk and feels a strong aversion to traditional medicine, so talking to her about my cancer was very unsettling to her. Still, her response was one of unconditional support for me, assuring me she would share the journey with me.

DAN

It would be harsh to say that Judy was determined to get cancer, and it would have been awfully callous to even suggest that once the diagnosis had been made. And while I never did make that observation at the time, I could not help that the thought crossed my mind. Obviously there was nothing factual to support such an idea, unless one believed in the mysterious dynamics of a self-fulfilling prophecy. Even that is a hard road to go down. It might be less severe, and possibly more accurate, to say that Judy had a long-running premonition that she was going to get cancer, and despite all her efforts to ward the illness off, it got her anyway.

There's a story of a man who comes face to face with Death (hooded robe, scythe, and all) outside his home in Oakland. Death raises its reaping tool, and the man jumps into his car and speeds away. He makes it to the airport, where he boards the first available flight. From the plane he calls his wife back in Oakland and tells her what has happened and that he is headed to Houston. His shaken wife goes outside the house and sees Death standing there. She walks up to the figure and asks why it had threatened her husband, hoping to somehow change destiny. Death said it had made no threatening gesture to her husband; the gesture was merely one of surprise. Death explained that it was startled to find her husband in Oakland, because it was scheduled to see the man later that day in Houston.

Judy had an appointment with cancer. It was something she knew was on her agenda. She didn't put it there; she didn't make the appointment. It was simply penciled into her inner day-timer a long time ago, already there when she started flipping ahead through the pages to see what lay in store for her. Though she tried in various ways and at various times to cancel the appointment, in the end the inevitability of it won out. As Gene Wilder said in the movie *Young Franken-stein*, "Destiny. Destiny. No escaping destiny." Cancer may not have been my personal bogeyman, but it certainly was hers.

I suppose a lot contributed to this unfounded—and what to me seemed unnatural—fear. For one, she had this zero-sum philosophy about the good and bad things life handed out to her. She saw life as a scale, a double-entry ledger that would always eventually be brought into balance. She believed that she had to pay for all the positives of her life. I first became aware of her belief in that rule one Sunday morning when a stranger knocked on our door and, out of breath, told me that Judy and Alex had been in a car accident. He described the car—Judy's car—and we quickly went the few blocks back to the accident scene. Neither Judy nor Alex was seriously hurt, though from the look of the car things could have been much worse. Judy rode in an ambulance to get checked out further at the hospital, while Alex and I followed in my car. In the emergency room she admitted to me that, "Things were going too good. Something like this was bound to happen." It was a CPA's approach to life: don't expect to accumulate too much good; the universe—or the IRS—will conspire to bring you back into balance.

Both of Judy's parents died of cancer, as did her grandmother. Cancer certainly seemed to be in her lineage. I assumed she was like me in that she looked to her family when she pondered how she might die. Dying wasn't something that she would dwell on, but everyone likely gets around to wondering how it will all eventually end, even those of us who, like me, remain convinced we are destined for immortality. When I forget that special designation, I figure my end will result from an accumulation of nagging problems. Even though my mother had breast cancer, I do not see cancer as being the death of me. There's a fair amount of heart-related stuff on my family tree, though nothing specific enough or dramatic enough to lead me to believe I will not slowly fade away.

Judy, obviously, had a different vision for herself. Again, maybe it was a premonition. Maybe it was what she gleaned from her family history. Maybe it was just a genuine psychological fear of something out of her control taking over her body, leaving her helpless. Whatever planted the seed, the result was that she took steps to promote her health with the intent of preventing cancer. Those steps, diet and exercise especially, certainly contributed to her overall good health. Even some of the supplements she took arguably made her a healthier person. But when the diagnosis came—when the dust had settled and she had digested the immediacy of the judgment—she felt betrayed, that maybe she had been hoodwinked. All the steps, all the preventative measures had not altered the outcome. In the end it was still cancer. The fact that it was breast cancer, with its high survival rate, as opposed to other types of cancer, mitigated the impact only somewhat. Cancer of any kind was the worst possible news for her.

By the time of the diagnosis, breast cancer had become more prevalent in our lives. People we knew had gone through the experience and how they handled it would be part of what informed us as we faced our own journey.

Gina, a friend and co-worker of Judy's, was diagnosed with breast cancer at the very time her own mother was dying of brain cancer. We had socialized with Gina and her husband a couple of times. Gina came over for dinner by herself one night, shortly after her diagnosis. We learned two things about Gina that night. One was that she was going to overwhelm her cancer with knowledge and willpower. That was her style. She would learn everything there was to know about the disease and all the treatment options, and she would put together a plan that would win the day. That plan involved conventional Western approaches along with less conventional methods, among them altering her diet. The other thing we learned was that, from her perspective, her husband was not going to be much of a help in the process. She would have to work around him. Gina relied more on friends and relatives, which resulted in Judy accompanying her to at least one chemo treatment, and though she did lose her hair (actually, she shaved it off before it could fall out), she never seemed to lose her composure. She went through her own treatment and her mother's death with as much strength and individualism as was always her nature.

About the same time, through some work contacts, Judy had been invited to join an afternoon book club. One of the members, Cathlin, was a breast cancer survivor. When Cathlin decided to produce a documentary film about breast cancer, Judy hooked her up with Gina. The documentary aired on public television. I remember it being a powerful piece, and years later, after Judy's diagnosis and after Cathlin died, Judy obtained a copy of it. Though we have not yet watched it again, it sits on the shelf waiting for the right moment for us to revisit it.

In addition to cancer experiences with friends and family, I had my own brief worry over it. Given Judy's ongoing fear of cancer, there is a certain irony in my having to deal with it first. At my first physical after turning fifty, a physical I delayed a couple of years, the doctor expressed some concern over the size and feel of my prostate gland, a concern that was confirmed by my blood work results. That led to seeing a specialist, which led to scheduling a biopsy. There was a lot of limbo time involved in that process. I had believed that if cancer was suspected, or was even a possibility, things should move fast to make that determination—or at least a little faster than they actually did. But I had to wait three weeks to see the specialist, and then the biopsy couldn't be scheduled for several weeks after that. I had a lot of time to think about "what if I do have cancer?" and how that might impact or alter what I was doing with my life.

This was all occurring at the time I was retiring from my twenty-five years in the hardware business. Retiring was a major decision, but not one I wanted to associate with illness. I was leaving by choice, not necessity. On the other hand, I had a bizarre curiosity about what it would feel like and be like to have an ongoing, life-threatening disease. I wondered how I would react, whether it would bother me that the disease would take my life's priorities and choices out of my hands. Pondering all this became an intellectual exercise, and my desire to know and experience living with a severe illness became strong. I have to admit to a definite degree of disappointment when I got word that my prostate was not cancerous. It was merely enlarged in a normal way, not inappropriate for my age. I participated in the ensuing relief and minor celebration, but a part of me was sorely disappointed. It was kind of like, "Nothing exciting ever happens to me." That's a pretty bizarre reaction, and I'm not sure I truly understand it, but I can't pretend I reacted otherwise.

I always seem to seek a different slant on things, and disease is no different. For example, I have always appreciated the disease-as-metaphor concept, wherein the symptoms reflect what is troubling the inner self, the soul. Taken on a grander scale, increases in the occurrence of certain kinds of diseases reflect how society and culture are negatively impacting individuals. Cholesterol-clogged arteries suggest the congested circumstances of modern metropolitan life. Similarly, fast-growing cancer cells mirror a fast-paced existence in which people rarely stop to take stock of the consequences of such a lifestyle until illness or accident forces them to. The problem with this metaphorical approach is that it adds blame—or worse, social commentary—to the stricken by suggesting it is a person's own fault, or society's, when that person gets ill. Adding the element of "why" or "why me" onto someone just diagnosed with cancer hardly seems worthwhile or fair. That person has enough to deal with, without delving into the philosophy of disease.

JUDY

In all the mental chaos following the diagnosis, my predisposition to panic and fear kept my mind from contemplating the obvious question—"Why me?" In fact, it was not until two months after my diagnosis that I got around to asking that question. The oncologist's reply was a straightforward, "Because you are a typical American woman."

Statistics confirm that. One out of eight women in the United States will develop breast cancer if they live past the age of eighty-five (a risk that in 1960 was one out of fourteen). I might have thought that my preventative measures gave me some dispensation, but such thoughts are nonsense. I was part of a large group of victims.

But I needed to move beyond thoughts of victimization and take stock of how I was going to endure the unpleasantness such a diagnosis entails. Even though my distinctive lifestyle hadn't prevented me from being victimized, I was hoping that the activities that I embraced would help me stay grounded.

To start with, I am my own boss. I work from home and do work that I love and believe in. After twenty-five years as a manager or program director in the nonprofit arena, I had identified a specialty area that allowed me to freelance and serve multiple clients at the same time. I am a writer and editor and assist non-profits in articulating and documenting their programs so that they can be as efficient and energized as possible in securing funding and in delivering their programs to their clients. The scope of projects I manage is pleasantly varied, and the stimulation of working in many different areas feeds my interest.

Being modest in my ambitions, I am content to work about twenty hours per week, which leaves me plenty of time to pursue a variety of other activities. At the time of my diagnosis I was happily involved with yoga, volunteer storytelling in two middle schools, working with a personal coach, dancing weekly with the local chapter of Dances of Universal Peace, getting monthly massages and Feldenkrais sessions, volunteer editing a professional organization's newsletter, walking a lot, and participating in three book clubs.

As I faced treatment, I wondered what activities I would choose to sustain, what new activities I would gravitate to, and what current activities I would drop off my list. I regularly chose things that were positive for my well-being, but would those things continue to be what I needed? What I felt capable of and interested in doing?

Of all my previous activities, I did sense that grandparenting would continue to be the most joyful. Spencer was only six months old when I was diagnosed, and we were fortunate enough to take care of him one day a week. Our granddaughter Maria was five years old and still fairly new to us, coming with our older son's new partner, but we were starting to see more of her. I didn't know how I would take to being a grandma before it actually happened, but once I became one I didn't need to grow into the role; I was a natural. There is something very exciting about being part of a developing life, something that occurs at a deeper level than it did when we were caring for our own children. As a grandparent I'm more mature, probably wiser, and much more aware of what I'm doing and what impact I'm making. Then there is the added benefit of getting to see the world through a child's eyes again and sharing the thrill of learning about life as if for the first time. What a treat. I knew that cancer might eventually interfere with that, but it also heightened my sense of the importance of each moment I got to spend with the grandkids.

Journaling became a new activity, starting on the day of my mammogram retake. I had always loved to write, and for many years writing took the form of correspondence to others. I have only used journaling in moments of self-doubt or frustration with others or when traveling. Now, as I faced the experience of cancer, I knew I needed an outlet for expressing the myriad of facts and feelings that would overwhelm me. I didn't necessarily write every day, and my journaling was always a mix of recording and reflecting. As I went through such deep changes, I recognized that it would be a service to myself to capture my experiences and thoughts in the moment. In that way, I could let them go from my mind at the time and still refer to them in the future as I became curious about what I had felt in the moment.

3

Decisions and Postdecisional Dissonance

JUDY

Once the core biopsy results proved positive, a sense of urgency settled in. I needed to meet with a surgeon, and—because like most people I didn't have a surgeon to call my own—I relied on the recommendation of my internist. I scheduled a consultation for the next day. We didn't know it then, but the surgeon would recommend an oncologist, a radiation oncologist, and a plastic surgeon. We would be meeting a lot of people in the coming weeks and making a lot of decisions.

Dr. Betsy Brew, the surgeon, began the consultation by re-explaining the mammograms and ultrasound. Then she presented the two basic surgical options: a lumpectomy with seven weeks of follow-up radiation, or a mastectomy, with the option of reconstructive surgery. In both cases, they would test lymph nodes, and if the cancer had spread, other treatments would be necessary. But she said, "Don't go there now." Before we left her office that first day, she told us the story of a previous patient whose worst complaint about her breast cancer experience was that it was "damned inconvenient." I believe Dr. Brew was setting the stage for what she hoped we would be saying in the near future. She sent us home with lots of reading material.

On the one hand, we were encouraged that the cancer was "caught early," evidenced by the fact that none of the medical professionals could even feel the lump. On the other hand, well, there wasn't really an other hand ... we didn't yet have enough information, but we still felt as if we were balancing between good scenarios and bad scenarios. Nothing was definite yet. We knew I'd have surgery to remove the one lump. There was another lump in the same breast that might also be cancerous or might be just a calcification. It needed to be tested. If it was benign, I could have a lumpectomy. If it wasn't, I would have a mastectomy. If I had the lumpectomy, I would have to have seven weeks of radiation. At the time, the thought of going for radiation five times a week for seven weeks sounded like a life sentence. I wasn't fearful of the treatments themselves, but the time commitment seemed overwhelming. It would keep me focused on my disease for seven additional weeks. I wouldn't be able to escape it.

So my initial response was to go ahead and get a mastectomy. In addition to eliminating the follow-up radiation treatments, I also would avoid the small procedure associated with testing that other lump. Get it all off of me. I reasoned that I'd rather have the peace of mind that it was all gone than the worry that something had been left behind. I know this may sound drastic to some, but when you suddenly hear you have a disease, your first instinct is to want to get rid of it, even if you aren't feeling any discomfort. So I cancelled an appointment with a radiation oncologist and scheduled one with the plastic surgeon to find out what reconstruction was all about.

Initially, I got so involved in exploring the option of plastic surgery that it turned out to be a welcome distraction. And a captivating one. In addition to reconstructive surgery, I could even get a reduction on the other breast. That sounded like a nice side benefit, or in the words of the plastic surgeon, it would "improve the saggy breast."

"Let's do it all," I thought, even though the plastic surgeon did say this decision was not like choosing between vanilla and chocolate but between prune and anchovy-flavored ice cream. "Neither is tasty," he reminded us. We listened to descriptions of the options, and we saw photos of the results of reconstructive surgeries. Then I was photographed in a thong as a "before" picture, and the doctor marked me up with a felt-tip pen to show where he would make the changes.

Dan was completely turned off by the visit with the plastic surgeon and the options he presented, but I was drawn to them. I wasn't really internalizing the information; when I found in my research that so many other people had opted for this choice, I felt it was, therefore, a good one for me. At that time I had not digested that the recuperation from reconstructive surgery would last a similar length of time as the radiation I was determined to avoid—and would also be a whole lot more uncomfortable. In hindsight, perhaps I was hypnotized—not literally, but figuratively. I would choose to undergo this extensive procedure, because then I would have paid my dues and be cured. It was a less than rational decision, but despite Dan's shock at a choice so drastic, we scheduled a mastectomy and reconstructive surgery for November 20. In doing so, I was focused on alleviating the worry factor and believed the more drastic the surgery, the better my chance for survival.

DAN

The day after the diagnosis, we met with a surgeon. I'm not sure who recommended Dr. Brew to us, but that person deserves a finder's fee. I was instantly comfortable with her, as was Judy, a first impression that remained true throughout the experience, even though we wound up seeing a lot more of her in the coming weeks than we would have preferred.

The situation, as presented by Dr. Brew, was pretty straightforward. The tumor had been detected early, and it was very small. The treatment alternatives were a lumpectomy followed by a regimen of radiation, or a mastectomy, with or without reconstructive surgery. Whether Judy needed chemotherapy was something that would be determined with an oncologist after the surgery and after the lymph nodes were inspected. The immediate concern was getting rid of the tumor.

I sat next to Judy as we listened to the options and knew exactly which one she was going to choose. We had been married for over thirty years and have been a couple since we were sixteen. While we have not yet grown to look alike, we have become so attuned to each other that it no longer surprises us when we discover we are thinking the exact thoughts at the same time. All of this contributed to my certainty that Judy would opt for the least invasive, quickest, over-and-done treatment that was offered: lumpectomy plus radiation. That would make the entire ordeal nothing more than the "damn inconvenience" Dr. Brew, quoting one of her patients, said it might be.

But I suppose that's why you still play the game—you never really know how it's going to turn out. There was no hesitation in Judy's voice when she told Dr. Brew to "just get rid of the whole thing." She didn't look to me for counsel or even for reassurance that I would support her decision. Her mind seemed made up ahead of time. Definitely a mastectomy. No question. And yet, even though I was surprised, looking back on the moment, it made perfect sense. It followed a logic I should have seen. I had presumed she would want the least treatment possible to be rid of the problem. I didn't take into account her long-established worry over cancer. Given that, overkill was the obvious choice. If you get rid of the entire breast, there will never be any concern over cancer coming back there again. And that was what motivated her decision.

But I think Dr. Brew was surprised as well. Lumpectomy and radiation seemed the more appropriate choice given the small size of the tumor and its early detection. She told us there was no hurry to make the decision. (Again, as with my prostate episode, we saw no sense of urgency from the medical community. Where did we get the idea that when cancer was involved, time was of the essence?) But since another procedure, a calcification biopsy, must be done if Judy chose the lumpectomy route, that procedure was scheduled for the following week (which Judy later cancelled since she was leaning so strongly to the mastectomy, rendering the biopsy superfluous). In the meantime, Dr. Brew gave us some reading material and the name of a plastic surgeon who would discuss the various reconstruction options with us.

After we left Dr. Brew's office, I expressed my surprise to Judy about her decision. "Well, hold onto your hat," she said, "because what I have to tell you now will really blow you away." Then she told me she wanted to go the reconstruction route. She was right—I was flabbergasted. I began wondering how well I really knew this woman. I realized some changes would be inevitable in this cancer journey, but I didn't expect the essential, core Judy, the one I had known for so long, to undergo such drastic changes so quickly. Still, mastectomy and reconstruction was a viable option, and I had neither the experience nor the specialized knowledge to argue against her choice. I had my intuition and my preferences. I also had the sense of what I would do for myself if the situation were reversed. It was at that point, when I considered what would be right for me, that I realized she was basing her decisions on her own innate sense of what was right for her. Under like circumstances, I would want and expect to be supported for following my own instinctive sense of what to do. Once I was able to appreciate that, I cancelled any further debate and simply asked that she assure me she was certain of her decision. When she did that, all I had to do was give her my unwavering support. Easy enough, considering what she would be going through.

A few days later we met with the plastic surgeon—actually *reconstructionist* sounds better to me, post–Civil War history notwithstanding. Plastic surgery often has a frivolous connotation attached to it, making the term out of place given the purpose of our appointment. But even when I thought of him as a reconstructionist, I must admit I did not care for the man. The word "sleazy" comes to mind, and the work he did, which I'm sure he did very well, conjured up images from a freak show. And to top it off, the process he described for reconstructing the breast, along with the possibility of having to reduce the size of the other breast to make them match (but he could only promise approximately), seemed a bit primitive and seat-of-the-pants. Not to mention the extended recovery and rehabilitation time. Naturally I kept all my thoughts about the doctor to myself and confined my remarks to assuring myself that Judy understood exactly what she was signing up for. She said she understood the procedure and was sure about undergoing it, so, even though I remained skeptical of the plan and unconvinced that Judy fully grasped all of its implications, a mastectomy and reconstruction operation was scheduled. The earliest both doctors' schedules could accommodate the joint operation was in three weeks.

JUDY

After the consultations with the surgeon and the plastic surgeon, there was time for thinking. Our medical professionals were eager to get us as much information as we needed about the options for treatment, but they all told us that we now needed to take our time in deciding what to do. What to do?! My gosh, if these experts didn't tell us exactly what to do, how could we, as lay people, make good decisions? But, fortunately, the time interval did allow me to revisit the choices I had made.

I used the time to talk to people who were not medical professionals. I chose to talk to people I knew who had had breast cancer, and especially those who had dealt with it recently. With treatments advancing so quickly, it didn't seem helpful to talk to people whose breast cancer experiences were anything other than recent. Those I spoke with were candid in sharing details of their experiences, and that helped me understand both the medical procedures as well as the potential emotional impact of each.

I talked with Paula, a childhood friend whose family had a history of breast cancer and who, in her midforties, had elected a prophylactic double-mastectomy along with reconstructive surgery. Paula empathized with my enthusiasm for getting it all off. She also gave me a reality check about the reconstructive surgery. Yes, the plastic surgeon had provided the details of the surgery, but when I heard from someone who underwent the procedure, I began to realize that it was much more invasive than I had originally thought and required a lengthy recuperation. It involved what the plastic surgeon had referred to as a trans-flap procedure, but I hadn't really grasped that it meant using abdominal tissue to create the new breast. According to Paula, the recuperation from the actual mastectomy was mild compared to the recuperation from the reconstruction. Another person confirmed this for me, and in fact said she had some regrets about her choice. She said during her recuperation her new breast felt as though it weighed three hundred pounds, because it felt attached to her abdomen muscles. She also had a scare when the reconstruction tissue showed signs of dying.

I talked to other women who had had lumpectomies and chemo, or lumpectomies and radiation, or mastectomies with chemo and radiation. I began to see other possibilities.

Then, on the recommendation of Dr. Brew, we rescheduled our appointment with the radiation oncologist, Dr. Kevin Schewe. Dr. Brew wanted us to fully understand all the options. By the end of the visit with Dr. Schewe, I doubted my earlier decision to go through with the more intensive procedure. He told us that recurrence happens in only 1–4 percent of women who choose lumpectomy and radiation. That sounded very positive. He said, "Seven weeks of radiation may sound like a lot now, but in the big picture of life, it's not a lot." The recovery from mastectomy with reconstructive surgery would be about six weeks, most of that recovering from the reconstruction. We cancelled the November 20 procedure. This is what is called a flip-flop in current political jargon; in medical jargon it was a flip-flop on the trans-flap.

But before we could schedule the lumpectomy, I had to have the second lump tested. If the calcifications were identified as precancerous, my initial decision to have it all taken off would hold. If the calcifications were benign, we would opt for the lumpectomy and radiation. That test was done on November 7, and, happily, the pathology came back "negative." I rescinded the decision to "do it all" and did a one-eighty on my earlier decision by deciding to go with a lumpectomy and sentinel node dissection, surgery option one.

DAN

Once the joint mastectomy and reconstruction surgery was scheduled, I think Dr. Brew decided to become a little more proactive in influencing what she thought was an under-considered decision on our part. I strongly sensed that was her motivation when she contacted Judy and persuaded her to at least meet with the radiation oncologist, Dr. Schewe. She wanted us to understand all the options before going ahead with the more extensive procedure. When we met with Dr. Schewe, he did not try to talk us out of our choice, but he did present us with enough statistical evidence to make Judy more comfortable with the idea of the lumpectomy and radiation route. With the numbers he presented, both treatments—lumpectomy and mastectomy—offered comparable degrees of certainty that the cancer would be gone and unlikely to return. And what Judy was beginning to process was that if the more difficult mastectomy offered no significantly better warranty, the "easier" option was more attractive.

So the calcification biopsy, which needed to be done before a lumpectomy could be a viable option, was rescheduled for the following week, still two weeks before the mastectomy/reconstruction appointment. It was an outpatient procedure requiring only a local anesthetic. After initially getting geared up for a more major surgery, we were by then equally eager to avoid it. So the outcome of that biopsy was going to do more than just inform; it was going to impact us emotionally. The wrong outcome would be a disappointment, leading us to more concerns and, maybe worse, more decision points. We were ready for something that was both positive and simplifying, something that put a definitive time limit on our journey. And that is exactly what we got.

Unlike the initial biopsy, which was done in the breast care center affiliated with the hospital, this second procedure took us to the outpatient surgery department of the hospital itself. That was not a problem, but it did offer some contrasts, primary among which was the emphasis away from nurturing to logistics (keeping the schedule) and verifying that the insurance and co-pays were in order. Of course, all those distractions and disappointments quickly disappeared when Judy and I found ourselves waiting in the preop room wondering about the procedure and what next steps we were facing.

The pathology report came back negative, which under the circumstances is the positive outcome, and Judy immediately cancelled the more major surgery, opting for the lumpectomy. Its minimal invasiveness, easier recuperation, and same long-term prognosis made it a no-brainer—a no-brainer that elicited a concealed sigh of relief from me. It took a while, but Judy and I were finally where I always sensed we should be, but more importantly, we seemed to be back on the same page. It's just that I forgot Judy had to do a little extra reading to get caught up. Judy was going through an additional thought process when making these decisions, needing to incorporate her long-term worry about cancer into all the other immediate factors involved. I was considering the other factors but not understanding the emphasis I needed to give the "Judy and her fear of cancer" factor. From that point on, we were back in sync. Functioning as a team again. And just in time.

4

What Are the Odds of Going Full Circle?

JUDY

On November 20, I wrote:

What will life be like after surgery? We don't know what we will find, but I want to be optimistic that the worst has already been discovered. Then we will heal. Then we will commence the regimen of radiation, which will require another commitment—disruption in the routine, physical impact, and opportunity to make everything else in my life more important, more enthusiastic, more appreciative, and more joyous. A hurdle is to be sailed over, with practice of course, but with confidence first and foremost. And then to look back and feel an incredible sense of accomplishment and awe in one's abilities. Why not? The alternative does not appeal.

I marvel at this confidence as I read back on it.

DAN

We were still a couple of months away from first hearing the roller-coaster metaphor applied to the cancer journey, but it was at this point that the ride really began. When the diagnosis was pronounced, we got our tickets and stepped into the car. Digesting all the information and making decisions was the long, slow pull up the first hill. The first surgery, the lumpectomy, was the release into free-fall, taking us to incredible low points only to be rocketed skyward again for a brief instant before the next plummet signaled a new cycle. The roller-coaster metaphor proved to be a great way to conceptualize our experience, except at the time we were unable to conceptualize much of anything. We were months away from appreciating the aptness of a metaphor. Metaphors require perspective, and perspective requires some distance. Being right in the midst of it all, we couldn't appreciate the analogy and really didn't have the time to even consider it. Instead of noticing the roller coaster, we were suddenly preoccupied with higher mathematics.

Welcome to the world of statistics and probability. Cancer, the logic seemed to be, is not so frightening and imposing when it is reduced to a series of numerical percentages and odds. All our health care providers must have attended a very convincing seminar during their schooling on how best to discuss the disease with a recently diagnosed patient. Or maybe they all read the same journal article on the subject. The reality was that all discussions concerning Judy's cancer with a medical professional involved—and then revolved around—a heavy dose of numbers.

I understand the doctor's dilemma. A newly diagnosed person will want, and need, to deal with the cancer emotionally. From the patient's perspective, who better to do that with than the doctor? Newly diagnosed cancer patients will want to hear not just reassuring, positive news, but they will also want guarantees and certainties. They don't want to hear "maybe" or "we'll see" or the dreaded "I don't know." However truthful that noninformation may be, it offers no calming effect. It actually adds frustration and anger and diminishes confidence in the entire health care profession. "How can they not know?" the patient wonders. Obviously such situations, involving a disparity between the patient's desire for a definite answer and the provider's inability to provide one, are painful for both sides—and unproductive.

The solution: don't even go there. Don't try to discuss the unknown. Instead, journey into the world of, "This is what we know for sure. Based on all recorded cases, X percent of patients diagnosed with your type of cancer survive and remain cancer free for the next Y years. With a regimen of chemotherapy and/or radiation, that success rate increases by Z." The beauty of the numbers racket is that it allows nothing messy in an emotional or interpersonal way. "These are the facts, ma'am. Just the facts." And then it is left to the patient to sense how one fits into the statistics, whether to extract optimism or become resigned to the worst-case scenario. The medical professional does not have to get involved in awkward emotional interactions, which can be a horrifically draining process if dealing with cancer is what one does for a living. By avoiding those entanglements, the health care provider can concentrate on what he or she knows best, which is providing the health care service.

JUDY

Dr. Brew did not overwhelm us with numbers the first time around. What we took from our initial consultation with her was that the tumor was small and it was detected early, and that this might prove to be just a "damn inconvenience." Implied in all that were pretty good odds that we'd be looking back on this scare with a light heart in a few months. That was a good thing to hear, just what we needed at the time.

And then Dr. Schewe used statistics to convince us that the lumpectomy-radiation route was statistically as effective as the mastectomy route. That, too, was good information at just the right time. The numbers were falling into place so far.

After checking in at the outpatient surgery desk for my lumpectomy, I returned to the breast center for a needle/dye procedure that would pinpoint where Dr. Brew was to operate. The only tense moment came when the technician told me they were going to take another mammogram. They had just put wires in my breast, and now they were going to squish it? That sounded tortuous, but they assured me that it would be fine. I trusted them, and, fortunately, they did not disappoint me. It was one of those moments that primed me to feel confident about putting myself in the hands of others.

Surgery is not supposed to be a walk in the park, but our hospital did offer some amenities to make it less scary, more comforting. And we took advantage of those amenities. We had a preop room that was quiet and calm, with low lights, music, a lavender-scented eye pillow, and purple blankets. Everyone who came into the room talked in a quiet voice—it is amazing what low lights can do to calm usually strident hospital voices. The nurse came in to introduce herself and to describe how I would be positioned in the OR. She was followed by the anesthesiologist, who was also an acupuncturist. Having had prior experience with acupuncture, I had opted for its use here to reduce the quantity of anesthetic and also to reduce the time needed to come out of anesthesia. These details mattered a great deal to us, and they relaxed both Dan and me. The only thing that reminded me of past hospital experiences was the difficulty the nurse had in starting the IV. I have a history of that, and it followed me to this situation; that was the worst part of the ordeal.

Surgery number one (November 21) was uncomplicated and was performed without incident. Dr. Brew's postop feedback was that everything looked good. She told us that the initial pathology results were 95 percent accurate, so when we went home the next morning, we felt relieved and optimistic. My focus was on the physical therapy exercises I had been instructed to do to regain 100 percent movement in my arm. I wrote in my journal the next day, *I geared up for the absolute worst, and now that it is the absolute best it feels like I only had a minor sliver after being threatened with a broken finger. How to put this in perspective?*

Then Dr. Brew's call came a few days later and deflated our bubble and introduced us to a new and foreign vocabulary. "The margins weren't good," she said, which meant the areas around the part that was removed indicated cancerous activity. I would need to have a re-excision to try and get margins that were free of cancerous activity—to be sure all the cancerous tissue was removed. The pathology on the lump was "ductal invasive carcinoma 1.1 cm, Grade III." Ductal invasive carcinoma means that the cells have left their original location and "invaded" the surrounding breast tissue. The size (1.1 cm) was small, but Grade III meant the type of cancer was aggressive (with Grade IV being the most aggressive). Grade is determined by appearance of the cells (the more they look like normal tissue, the lower or better the tumor grade) and occurrence of division (the fewer the number of cells dividing, the lower the tumor grade, because the slower the tumor is likely to grow). The pathology on the sentinel node was "micrometastatic carcinoma .2 cm," meaning the cancer had spread beyond the breast. Given Grade III pathology and the spread into the lymph nodes, chemo became the likely treatment. *We celebrated too soon. The final pathology report does not agree with the initial one—we are in the 5 percent in which that happens. Damn it! What a horrible letdown.*

After that, I felt as if I turned my calendar over to Dr. Brew's scheduler, Cindy. We talked frequently, and not just about scheduling. I called her for anything related to my cancer, like when I panicked and thought Grade III was the same as Stage III. When you are suddenly overwhelmed with medical data, it is very easy to go off the deep end, to become confused, and to activate the panic gene. And also to grab on to these medical terms as describing you in a new way.

I knew the higher the stage, the more serious the cancer. Cindy explained to me that grade and stage mean different things, and that the stage of my cancer was not III. Stage depends on the size of the tumor and the spread of the cancer: the higher the stage, the more extensive and serious the cancer. There are five stages, 0 to IV. With a positive pathology on my lymph node tissue, my cancer indicated early Stage II. With earlier technology, that same tissue would have given a negative reading, indicating Stage I. Very small cancers, like mine, are now able to be detected but have probably not existed long. Grade III has fast-growing cells that are not at all like normal cells. This would explain why a small tumor had already gotten into the lymph node.

Cindy, like most everyone else we encountered during my illness, was very professional and very helpful. We just preferred not to be in a position of needing help. But given that we did, we felt very fortunate in our choice of doctors. We came to them through the initial referral from my regular doctor, not through any research on our own part. We simply trusted the fates in that regard. That the surgeon we were first referred to was so much to our liking gave us confidence. I can't imagine what going through all this might have been had we struggled with finding good doctors.

I am very trusting when it comes to working with people who are professionals in their fields. I respect their training and commitment, and I believe they have strong ethics and my best interests at heart when they work for (or on) me. I've never had an experience to suggest otherwise. So when it came to dealing with cancer, I relied on the cancer professionals. I believed and followed their advice and was content and confident in what they proposed. That is not typical, I think. Many people are more cynical than I about the perfection (or adequacy) of who they deal with and are more curious to explore other options—the more options the better. I am always overwhelmed at the thought of exploring other options, and I choose not to go there. I figure that my belief system has a lot of power to affect the outcome of my care, and I choose to invest those beliefs in thinking the best of those responsible for my care. Throughout this journey I looked to my health care professionals to have the answers and to meet my needs, and I was never shy about expressing those needs.

We loved our doctors, and we believed in them. In fact, only one person in the medical arena offended me during my treatment. She was a volunteer with the hospital's cancer support group. She meant well, and she had experienced what I was going through, but I could not abide her. She barged into the needle/dye procedure I had at the breast center to present me with a breast cancer pin; the technicians thought she must have been my mother or mother-in-law to have assumed such authority. I saw her again in the radiation facility, schmoozing with radiation patients, getting in their face with her story and asking about theirs. Perhaps it speaks to the support riches I already had, but I did not want her support. She drained me. I was nice enough to her but never encouraging. It seems silly that a patient should have to fend off an offer of support. When it came time to consider support groups, there was never one moment when I considered going to the support group she led. Given all that I was dealing with, I probably was ultrasensitive to what I considered her abrasive style. (And this paragraph will be the only paragraph in this entire memoir that is critical of an offer of assistance.)

DAN

The day of the lumpectomy came. Judy had arranged for the upgrade treatment, meaning we got a private preop room that came with soft lighting, a TV/VCR setup in case we wanted to bring something to watch while we waited, a stereo so we could listen to the music of our choice, and acupuncture-assisted anesthesiology. It was as pleasant as it could be, like getting bumped into first class on an otherwise tedious flight. Except that when the time in preop was over, Judy was still wheeled off to the operating room, and I was relegated to the general waiting room.

It seemed I waited a long time, yet the time was neither peaceful nor reflective, as I had anticipated. Instead I found it a trying, annoying wait, beset with constant intrusions into what I had hoped would be some private space in which I could contemplate the magnitude of what was going on in the operating room. It was difficult to find a spot in the waiting room where I did not have to watch television. TVs seemed to be everywhere, and on, and loud, and all with a cadre of captive viewers, choosing to lose themselves in any daytime fare when they weren't talking on their cell phones. The only television-free space was right in front of the reception desk, where instead of a talk show or a soap opera, I had to endure the too-candid banter of the reception staff, the too-personal details of those checking in for surgery, or the too-impatient queries of those who felt they had waited long enough and demanded to be told what had gone wrong with their loved one's operation. Everyone seemed to irritate me, and yet I could not block anyone or anything out. I changed seats a lot, and after about two hours of waiting, I finally outlasted a group around a television set, which, once the area was vacated, I turned off. I then readied myself to snap at anyone who dared to come along and try to turn it back on.

I didn't get the chance to enjoy the peace for long. Dr. Brew came out to tell me that everything went well and that the preliminary look at the tissue made her 95 percent certain they got it all. Verification would come on Monday. It was Friday afternoon. Judy would be in recovery for a while and then would get a room upstairs for the night. I could see her when she was settled into the room. Until then, I just had to wait.

I took that time to pull out my list of phone numbers and begin making calls, reporting the successful and optimistic news. I called our sons first. Both were relieved at the news, and both would come to the house the next day to be with Judy while I squeezed in some hours at work. Next I called Judy's sister Laurie. Laurie was the relay person for the other sisters, Debbie and Bonnie. Laurie was also a nurse, so once I assured her that Judy was fine and the operation was a success, she dragged all the details out of me regarding the more technical aspects of it, as if I knew what I was talking about. Our good friends Mary and Gail were next on the list, and both were happy and relieved at the report. And grateful. That confused me a bit. Grateful at the news, or grateful I had called them? I wasn't sure. I told each of them, "You've been a close friend for a long time. You're important to us, to Judy. We're grateful to *you*."

It was a good and grateful weekend that, like all weekends, ended on Monday. And when that particular Monday came around, we were informed that the long shot had come in. We fell outside the 95 percent certainty of good news. The margins were not clear, meaning the tissue around the tumor that was removed was not cancer free. A re-excision would have to be done. The pathology report also indicated that chemotherapy would likely be part of the subsequent treatment, since the cancer had spread to the lymph nodes. Dr. Brew explained that the procedure is imprecise, and a surgeon can only remove what experience has shown to be enough to yield a clear margin. In most cases, one surgery takes care of things, but having to do a re-excision is not unusual.

"Most" does not correlate to a specific percentage, but the message was that we just happened to draw the short straw. We were a wee bit unlucky. It was not the first time things didn't go as perfectly and as smoothly as we had planned or hoped, but none of the previous occasions measured up to the import of this one. Breaking my foot the week before a long-anticipated vacation or being sued by the people who bought our house were the worst possible eventualities when they occurred, but they seemed trivial now. They were anecdotes we would never tell again, because they suddenly lacked the key ingredient to their impact—they no longer had anything at stake. It seemed that all memories of disappointment and frustration and bad luck from that point on would have to be measured against hearing that one surgery wasn't enough, that the surgeon had to go back in and cut out some more of Judy's breast.

I'm not sure how we managed the in-between time. I had work to fill up part of the days, and fortunately my work was of the type that required all my concentration. It is detailed work, and the pace is just frenetic enough that the bulk of my day flies by without allowing me to think about anything else. But, at the same time, my work doesn't leave with me when I punch out for the day. Judy, working from home, must have found it more challenging to occupy her time and her thoughts during the interval before the second surgery. I always finished up work and got home as quickly as I could to be with her, especially if she had no appointments that day.

JUDY

What to do when one waits? And what is one waiting for? Should I be wait-ing—should I go out and meet it more directly? I feel like I need more structure in my days—definitely getting out more. My mind is not feeling very creative at the moment—I'm in a mood of self-pity. Should I curl up in bed or go out for a walk? I will have this choice every day.

Surgery number two was scheduled for December 4, two weeks after the ini-tial lumpectomy. The surgeon removed additional breast tissue and installed a chemo port. We tried to remain optimistic and upbeat. And we took every opportunity to be playful. In the recovery room after the surgery, Dan was trying to give me some juice to drink. When I leaned forward and met him halfway, he pulled the straw away from me. He repeated this routine several times. Then when he decided he had had enough fun, he fed me pudding, which I took, though I was sorely tempted to purse my lips and give him a raspberry. Funny how his mouth would open as he put the spoon in mine! It felt absolutely won-derful to laugh so hard—the best medicine, bar none.

The postsurgery info followed a disappointingly familiar pattern: encouraging results immediately and a deflating phone call a few days later. "Extensive lym-phatic involvement by poorly differentiated ductal carcinoma Grade III," mean-ing there were cancerous cells in my breast's lymphatic vessels. Dr. Brew said she had never seen anything like this before, a statement which at face value was not very reassuring. She meant that she hadn't ever seen cancer cells in this early a stage; she sees them after they have progressed for a while. I wrote in my journal, *Do you believe how badly every procedure has gone? Well, not the procedure exactly, but the pathology gleaned from the procedure. Do I have to describe how cut off at the knees I felt again with this round of bad news? Just beat up, numb in some ways, just tragic in all ways.*

The disappointment after the first surgery and the realization that chemother-apy would be necessary was bad enough. Somehow this latest blow was worse than the first, maybe because it established a pattern of something unexpectedly going wrong. And we still needed to move forward. There was no time to do oth-erwise. No choice. We were oh-so-eager to take every option that would make good news a possibility again.

A mastectomy now became the recommended procedure. So here we were fac-ing what I had chosen initially. The 180-degree turn this time was not voluntary, but now I was very clear that there would be no reconstructive surgery. Enough surgery already. At fifty-five I knew I could adjust to an asymmetrical torso and a prosthesis. As I wrote that day, *I didn't have strong feelings about losing a breast—I wanted it off because it was no longer healthy or happy. I would work to have an outward appearance that was "normal," but I was sure I wouldn't feel terrible looking for what wasn't there anymore.* I did inquire whether we should also have the right breast removed. The surgeon and medical oncologist said that was not necessary.

DAN

The time did eventually pass, and two weeks later, also on a Friday, we were back at the hospital.

Our son Darren joined me in the waiting room that day. Rather than staying there the entire time, we went to the hospital cafeteria to get something to eat. After returning to the waiting room, we had only a short wait before Dr. Brew came out to see us. The report was pretty much the same as the first time. Judy was doing fine, the operation went well, and the preliminary look left the doctors 95 percent sure they got it all, pending verification on Monday. We stayed around until Judy was out of recovery and situated in a room. We visited with her for a while, but it soon became clear that she was more worn out than after the previous surgery—or, more likely, she just wanted to take advantage of the lingering anesthetic and get a deep, untroubled rest. Darren and I left her that afternoon, and I returned alone for a brief visit that evening. I was back the following morning to take her home.

The pathology report again came on a Monday, with the same disappointing results as two weeks before. We had beat the odds again. The cancer was more aggressive than initially thought, more aggressive than anything Dr. Brew said she had experienced before, considering how small the cancer was when it was detected. The upshot of the pathology was that a mastectomy was the only recommended next step.

A mastectomy? Wasn't Judy's initial gut reaction to have a mastectomy and "just be rid of it"? There is something to be said for following one's instincts. After all the consultations and consideration of the options, after all the processing of statistics and odds, after two biopsies and two surgeries, we were still not out of the first phase of dealing with Judy's cancer. The frustration was persistent and almost all-consuming, but I think, if nothing else, we had an appreciation of just how much is not known about cancer and how much it varies from person to person. There are no hard and fast rules—at least not yet. That's why all the push for research dollars. That's why they have events like Race for the Cure. Understanding that helped stave off the frustration, but that was not the only thing weighing on our minds.

In fact, it is probably accurate to say that we were less disappointed by the pathology report after the re-excision than we were by the bad news we received with the lumpectomy. This time we weren't just fretting over bad luck and the prospect of more surgery. What replaced all that and what made the next step easier to accept was alarm. What jumped out of this second pathology report, and what redefined everything, was that Judy's cancer was aggressive. That's a tough word to deal with. It has a lot more implications than we had been dealing with to that point. We were still fixated on the "damn inconvenience" of it all and, frankly, didn't want to give that up. Calling it an aggressive cancer changed all that. The fact that it was aggressive led me to wonder what might have happened if Judy had not been so diligent and compulsive about cancer, which had compelled her to check for it so religiously. But that kind of wondering was for a larger perspective at a later time. We were faced with the immediacy of what that word *aggressive* implied, and that meant getting rid of the cancer. And this time with not even a moment's consideration to reconstruction. That seemed trivial when *aggressive* was involved.

Looking back, I am sure deep down we understood that when we opted for the least invasive, easiest treatment option, we were playing the odds. All the numbers we heard indicated that the lumpectomy followed by radiation was as close to a sure hand as we were going to get in this game. When a sure thing fails to materialize, there may be a moment or two when regret or blame tries to mitigate the disappointment. But eventually one has to get around to wondering about destiny. Why didn't the great master plan allow for our situation to play out as such circumstances usually play out? Instead, our fate seemed to be riding the roller coaster. We couldn't even address *why* at the time. We were so caught up in the urgency of the events as they were unfolding that pondering the message in all of this would have to wait for a bit.

The mastectomy was scheduled for December 12.

5

Balancing a New Figure

JUDY

I sound almost cavalier about losing a breast, and I can understand how appalling that may seem. But I am very pragmatic and refuse to spin despair when I know it's not the best option. (Well, yes, I did spin despair in that childhood experience of thinking a mouth sore was cancer … I guess my pragmatism didn't come until adulthood.) The best option in the current circumstance left me eager to be rid of my breast. It held no special attachments for me; I had no strong, nostalgic entanglements with it, nor was it an integral part of my identity and self-esteem as a woman. It was dispensable, something that needed to be left behind if I were to move forward.

The truth is that my history with my breasts was not one of total adoration. I developed early and I am short. From the age of thirteen, I felt out of proportion and self-conscious about my breasts. Wearing swimsuits in my teen years made me even more self-conscious. I envy those young women today who appear to take greater pleasure in being amply endowed and who are not self-conscious, who even wear clothes that accentuate their endowments. I usually sought to minimize and cover up my breasts. So when we initially talked about reconstructive surgery and the plastic surgeon offered a reduction on the remaining breast, I got excited, picturing myself more comfortable with my chest.

While greater comfort was appealing, I wasn't seeking to achieve what the media tells us is a perfect figure. I really take pride in things about me for which I can take responsibility and credit, like my mind, my personality, and my accomplishments. I view my breasts as just part of the body equipment that I am genetically predisposed to have.

I have taken pleasure in being touched on my breasts and I know my loving husband has an affinity for them, but I didn't fear that I would be seen as lacking without one of them. The rest of me was still intact.

Many (probably most) women enjoy the pleasure of breast-feeding their children, and I envy them. I didn't have a strong desire to breast-feed my children and in fact inherited my mother's attitude, which was that it was difficult; therefore, I was not successful at it. In today's culture, with its greater appreciation and accommodation for breast-feeding, and the many resources that assist women in succeeding at breast-feeding, I expect I would have a more positive experience. I knew that breast-feeding reduces the risk of breast cancer ... but that was one preventative tool I had not used. And not one to dwell on at this point.

Would looking at a lopsided chest the rest of my life freak me out? Would I be continually reminded that I had had cancer? At the point of contemplating the mastectomy, and knowing it was the best option, I didn't think I would be freaked out, and I didn't think my breast's absence would continually remind me that I had had cancer. Humans have an incredible resiliency and ability to adjust to such seemingly catastrophic losses. I remembered Lois Hjelmstad revealing her double-mastectomy scars on the front page of the *Colorado Woman News* in the mid-1990s. It was the first time I had seen what a woman looked like after a mastectomy, and I actually kept that issue of the newspaper for a long time in my collection of interesting articles. When I saw Lois in person at the 2004 Day of Caring conference, she showed me a magazine article and photo of a group of women, including her. They were all baring their torsos—some with single mastectomies, some with double mastectomies. It was not frightening to me, just different. And yes, now I know that I probably will be continually reminded of my cancer, but that will be part of who I am; this experience revised my life story, and I am ever one to integrate individual experiences into my whole being.

DAN

There was a definite sense of relief in knowing that with the mastectomy this phase of the journey would finally be over. Certainly we were anxious about what was coming next and what we knew of chemotherapy did not make it something anyone would be eager to get into, yet we were. All we wanted at that time was to be out of the surgery phase. We didn't seem to be getting anywhere. Instead of positively progressing through a treatment regimen, Judy was facing her fifth surgical procedure in less than two months. We were gun-shy about always having our optimism shot down. So we embraced having the mastectomy done. Getting rid of the whole thing didn't seem to have any strings attached. Once it was gone, we could move on to the next step. Nothing else would be left to intervene.

Despite all the compelling reasons for the mastectomy, I did, understandably, take some time to ponder exactly what the "whole thing" was really about. The "it" that was being gotten rid of was Judy's left breast. It was a part of her body and a part of who she was. And while Judy had a more enduring claim on it, I certainly had a claim of endearment. That breast and I went back a long way. Not quite as long as my relationship with Judy, but it definitely was a significant part of the package that so attracted me, way back when. So while I didn't have any reservations or second thoughts about the decision to get rid of it, the reality and the permanence of doing so did warrant some heartfelt reflection and reminiscing, if not an outright eulogy. I couldn't let an old friend pass without saying a few words on the relationship we had shared.

On some long-forgotten occasion with another couple, perhaps on a double date, the discussion took a bizarre turn. Somehow we found ourselves discussing men's preferences for the various physical attributes of women. The discussion had not gotten very far when Judy stunned us by sitting up straight, sticking her chest out, and saying, "There's no guessing about what kind of man Dan is." It is true. With poultry I'm a leg man, all drumsticks and thighs, but when it comes to women, my heart and my eyes are drawn to the breasts. It's an appreciation thing, not a fixation, and I do quickly get around to other things, like mind and personality, etc. Judy, and our forty years together, will vouch for that; we wouldn't have lasted very long if I hadn't quickly started appreciating those other parts. So while the upcoming mastectomy might leave me a little traumatized and scarred, it was not going to be a threat to our relationship. Certain things would be different, but not insurmountable.

The fact that it was the left breast also presented no particular issue. Several weeks after the surgery, in another one of those bizarre discussions about body part preferences, Judy revealed to one of her sisters and a friend that I had always preferred the right breast anyway, so the loss, in that regard, was not so keenly felt. Not having heard that comment in person and therefore unable to ascertain the spirit in which it was made, I feel I must respond, as it contains the slightest innuendo that perhaps my neglect, or rejection, had a part in the left breast's demise. Not true. It just so happens that for the past ten years I slept on the left side of the bed, with Judy on my right. From that position, when I turned on my side to face Judy in moments of intimacy, it was my left hand that was most free, making her right breast most often the object of my attentions, or is it intentions? It was not favorites or preferences; it was logistics. I have slept on the left side of the bed because, in our most recent floor plan, it left me closest to the nearest facility, which I unfortunately have to get up and use more than once during a normal night's sleep (due to the enlarged prostate I mentioned earlier). Convenience put me there. And just to further clarify this and set the record straight, from 1970 to 1972 in our first apartment, and then from 1979 to 1995 in our southeast Denver home, I slept on the right side of the bed, meaning the same logistical conveniences had me predominantly attentive to her left breast.

That settled, I can't speak to how the prospect of losing a breast affected Judy. While there may have been a certain amount of nostalgia involved, I have to believe that any such feelings had long been cancelled out by the sense of her left breast having become more of a liability than an asset. Whatever part it had once played in her past persona, there was no role for it in her future. I don't believe she ever dwelt much on her femininity. She was always natural about such things and didn't spend a lot of time absorbed in the kind of thinking or the activities that went along with being a woman, or what culture defined as a beautiful woman. She just was one. Two breasts didn't make her who she was; having only one would not diminish her in any way. In her eyes, or in mine.

JUDY

Surgery number three (December 12) was my mastectomy. I remember few of the details. We waited in our special, dimly lit preop room, and I believe we were there a long time. For some reason, probably the sheer diversion of it, we were playing a game of naming as many beers as we could, along with their tagline or jingle. It must have been a compelling game, because when one of the technicians came in to do her routine "we haven't forgotten about you" checks, she helped us out as we struggled to remember an old-time jingle for one of the Wisconsin brews. We also listened to a selection from a friend's CD for children, appropriately titled "Itchy Itchy Owie Owie Boo Boo."

Eventually the waiting, and the fun, ended, and I was taken away to the OR. It was indeed the relief I had hoped and needed. I felt great as soon as I woke up from the anesthetic. No nausea, very little pain, and a lighter head and heart (and body, to be truly accurate). And this time, the pathology results indicated clear margins. Two additional lymph nodes were dissected and removed. They showed microscopic cancer. The mastectomy was the right decision.

And so the rounds of surgery were over. I felt relief. Even though they had not been horrible experiences, other than the pathology results, it felt good to finally have them over. Dr. Brew also expressed relief that she would no longer have to call us with bad surprises. I spent the night in the hospital. Again a physical therapist instructed me in the postsurgical exercises I would do for quite a while. Then, at home, I conducted a "throwing out the old bras" ritual. It was just something I came up with so I could let go of some of my frustration at having cancer. I blamed it on the bras. How easy it was to get rid of them! A symbolic letting go.

DAN

I anticipated a sorrowful farewell to Judy's left breast that day in the preop room, but it never really happened. We were too busy enjoying the moment and the music. Beausoleil was playing on the stereo. We passed the time trying to remember beer commercials, though I cannot recall how we ever got off on that tangent. I had prepared a farewell speech for the soon-to-be-departed—a few words to say thanks for all the moments together and for always being there when I was most in need. But when the time came and the nurse was about to push me aside so she could wheel Judy and her left breast off to the operating room, all I could think to say was, "Bye-bye, booby."

The surgery went well, and I left Judy in good spirits that night. I arrived at the hospital early the next morning, despite knowing it would be a few hours before Judy would be released. Dr. Brew and a physical therapist would have to see her, and she would have to pass all the other hospital checkout procedures before they let her go. We ate breakfast together—hers came with the room, mine from the cafeteria. While we were eating, Dr. Brew showed up. A relieved Dr. Brew. In the course of the lively and emotional conversation that followed, she revealed to us a sense of relief at having finally settled her portion of the Judy Gordon case. Thinking of her perspective, it could not have been pleasant to have two surgeries not be as successful as they initially seemed to be, and have to call us a few days after each one to undermine our relief by telling us we weren't done yet. But that morning we were done.

We arrived home to an assortment of children and grandchildren, and I left Judy with them while I headed off to work. It was already an established routine, having followed it three of the previous five Saturdays—a routine all of us were ready to give up. Everyone was optimistic and in good spirits.

I think it took a while for Judy to be comfortable with her altered physique. She stuffed socks into her empty bra cup to present a more balanced front to the world. We were told that she would not have any real sensation on her chest where the breast had been removed. She would feel pressure, but because the nerves would all be gone she would have no feeling. For a while she was careful to avoid much contact there, although every so often an overexuberant friend would give a close, hard hug that made her wince but also helped her realize she wasn't as fragile as she thought. The effects of the surgery, and the ugliness and disfigurement of it, slowly disappeared as she healed.

After coming to terms with her new look for herself, she next had to deal with going public. Some situations came up so suddenly that handling them was instinctive—like when she took grandkids Spencer and Maria swimming. They saw her when she dressed afterward and wondered why she looked different. Children may be too inquisitive and embarrassingly candid in places like a locker room, but they are also quite adaptable. So Judy's explanation to them was just one more thing about the world to learn and accept. A similar situation occurred when friends asked Judy to go to a local steam bath on ladies' night. When Judy expressed reservations about baring herself, her friends assured her there was nothing that had not been seen there already. That wasn't quite true. The night Judy went with them, one of the friends could not contain her curiosity and pointed to the button-shaped bulge high on Judy's right breast and asked what it was, having never seen a chemo port before. The encounter proved there was always something new to learn. It wasn't long after that that Judy decided it was too uncomfortable to try to look balanced when she exercised, so she started going to yoga classes lopsided.

It also took some time for me to feel comfortable touching her there, where her left breast had been. I purposefully avoided doing so at first, because I was afraid she still felt tender there. Later I avoided the area because I remembered she had no feeling there anyway. I guess I was concerned about how she might react emotionally to being unable to feel where she once had. Eventually, and it really didn't take all that long to get to the point, I decided it was too awkward to have a free right hand dangling in the air trying to be inconspicuous while my left hand was involved with her right breast. And just because the spot wasn't what it once had been did not mean it wasn't there, did not mean it wasn't a part of her. So I put my hand there now, and whatever she physically does or doesn't feel is unimportant compared to the message she receives in her head and in her heart: "No matter what, I still can't keep my hands, both hands, off you."

Two years after the mastectomy, we were at a play in a small theatre, sitting in the second or third row. A sign in the lobby had warned us that there would be nudity in the play, so it was not as if I was unprepared for what was coming. But when the actress pulled off her top and presented two large breasts to the audience, I was taken aback. Two of them? I marveled, stupefied, at the sight. It seemed so extravagant. And frivolous. Certainly ostentatious. And definitely redundant.

Adjusting is amazingly easy.

JUDY

Now we start putting some pieces back together again and preparing for the next challenge.

I used the time between surgery and treatment to reflect on all that had happened since my diagnosis and to try to gain some perspective. The focus of our thoughts, conversations, and actions from diagnosis day through the start of chemo two months later was the unwelcome world of medicine, of disease. We were meeting many medical professionals, all of whom we wanted to trust and from whom we wanted answers and assurances. We were consumed with procedural things. There is so much information to deal with. We needed to be thoughtful, inquisitive, and focused, and at the same time we still had our daily lives to maintain. But cancer creates chaos and confusion. Prospects are overwhelming when cancer is present in your life. Emotions surface quickly. Crying came easy to me, and I let it come. It washed over me. Sometimes I felt relieved, and sometimes I felt drained. But it always felt necessary. There were tears of fear, of frustration, of sadness, of prayer, and of being touched by others' care and concern. The tap was quick to flow; it was always primed.

Until we needed medical professionals, until I had breast cancer, health care providers and people with diseases were not in our daily lives; in fact, they were mostly invisible. Then we became immersed in that arena. And suddenly I couldn't imagine that I never knew the extent of people affected by disease, the continuum of care available, and the range of treatment options. I believe I read this in another person's cancer memoirs, and I felt this way, also: I so appreciated all the wonderful care I was receiving that my thoughts turned to how I could give back, how I could help others in this situation. It just seemed the most natural and heartfelt thing to pursue. As treatment became more routine, however, I began to take for granted the excellent care I was receiving, and my thoughts turned to other activities And perhaps I wanted people with disease and the whole health care system to become invisible again.

All the time that Dan and I were visiting with doctors and learning about my disease and its treatment options, we were sharing what we learned with my sisters and our two sons and their families. And we were candid with them, as we were with everyone. We shared what we knew, we shared how we felt. But we learned from our sons that they felt we were being too matter-of-fact in our conversations. Even though we shared information with them as quickly as we could, we had already processed our emotions by the time we told them what was going on. The way we communicated wasn't working for them. They told us that they needed us to keep our emotions current, to share not only on a factual level but on an emotional level. It was a good course correction, because we needed them to be as close to us as possible during this ordeal.

My sisters and I had had a different experience with our parents' illnesses, and I felt strongly that neither my mother's way nor my father's way would be *my* way. My father had not been feeling well when he was diagnosed with lung cancer and given six months to live; that was back in 1978, when hospice care was new. I believe we all benefited from the involvement of hospice, but Dad never progressed beyond the stage of anger, and we were young enough to have no idea what our own needs were or how we might best relate to him in his final days. My mother was the buffer and the manager who presented his status in the best possible light. He did die within six months.

When Mom was diagnosed with ovarian cancer in 1995, she vigorously pursued treatment but shared little about it with any of us. If we had had fewer demands in our own lives, perhaps we would have sought more conversation with her so that we could be fully present in her experience. She was stoic, however, and preferred to control the flow of information and the flow of emotions. Treatment worked for a couple of years, but when the cancer recurred in 1997 and she learned there were no further treatment possibilities, she resigned herself to dying. She felt that the quality of life she had known was gone. I believe she couldn't or didn't choose to define a new quality of life. While she appeared to engage in her favorite activities (going to the symphony, playing bridge, and being part of family events), she actually would have preferred to have died three months before she did. My sisters and I felt close to her physically but not emotionally. Our emotional experiences came from sharing with one another.

So it mattered to me that those around me during my cancer journey felt included. I believe people benefit from the truth, and I believe in being authentic to myself. I am a big sharer of information about myself, and just because this was not happy information (as most had been all my life), I didn't feel it was less important to share. Perhaps I even became a bit evangelical. I knew I felt better when people talked straight about things to me, and so I was taking my own role-modeling seriously. I would tell people how things were with me, no matter what was going on, and my candidness would demystify for them this whole cancer experience. Even in this day and age when we all know people who have or had cancer, knowledge is not widespread about the experiences of treatment, especially the emotional experiences.

I don't think I scared anyone away with my tell-all attitude. In fact, I heard from some people, after the fact, that they appreciated my candidness. They always knew how I was feeling and what I needed, and that made them feel more involved and appreciated. Telling my story allowed others to tell theirs (about self, friends, and loved ones). It opened the door to my accepting inquiries and support, and I was overwhelmed with cards and other messages. My diagnosis came just before the winter holiday season when we traditionally send personal messages to friends. This year was no different. True to our preferred communication pattern, we needed people to know what was actually going on with us.

I wrote and said this over and over again: *It feels good to share my story with loved ones. I need their support. I need to know they know what's really happening with me and that they can talk to me about what's going on … Thank goodness I am able to speak whatever it is I need to speak! I certainly could not put on a façade.*

It was people who had experienced cancer themselves who said the things that helped me the most. They were my role models, and I invested a lot in the lessons from their experiences. Someone three months ahead of me in treatment advised me to "just do it one day at a time." Paula, my childhood friend who had experienced breast cancer and subsequent prophylactic mastectomies, counseled me, "You just keep feeling better after a while, and then you forget how bad you had felt." Others told me, "You can get through it, and you will." They spoke of what they knew to be true. Their statements were not profound or revelatory, but they were real, and they resonated with me.

Others, who had not experienced cancer, also gave advice and support. I believe I valued this advice differently. I heard advice like "Don't give up your power," and "Keep yourself feeling in charge," and "Stay centered." After what I actually experienced, I would not advise others in this fashion. If I had to choose a simplistic way of expressing my advice, I'd say, "Be true to yourself in how you cope."

DAN

We saw Dr. Brew for a final checkup about ten days after the mastectomy. In the meantime we had met with the oncologist and were scheduled for Judy's first chemo treatment on December 22. We had received the diagnosis on October

22; it had only been two months. The roller-coaster ride had been so intense, we had lost track of time. The Race for the Cure event seemed like an eternity ago. We discussed all that with Dr. Brew and then told her that the date of the first chemo was significant in that it was the shortest day of the year. Things would begin getting sunnier after that. She liked that. We liked that. It was a good metaphor, positive and hopeful. It was also incredibly naïve. We thought we had been through the worst of things, and we were probably a little smug.

It is tempting to insert here the famous words about pride going before the fall, and perhaps to add a little anecdote to illustrate the point. But to do so would be to ascribe almost a divine intervention into the process, as if cancer, or cancer treatment, were the punishment for some heinous crime or personality defect. That's a little extreme, and even if it's true, I prefer not to know that the universe operates that way.

It is also tempting to incorporate a sports analogy about the mistake of taking an opponent too lightly or celebrating the victory too soon, while the race is still on or there is still time on the clock. But to do that personifies cancer as the evil enemy. The entire experience is then reduced to some morality play or melodrama in which everyone is but a caricature of good guy, bad guy, or victim. Life's more complex than that, certainly more intricate than a routine Hollywoodesque confrontation between good and evil. Things were dramatic enough without going that far. What happens on a personal and interpersonal level to ordinary individual human beings *is* the big stuff of life. That's what we were dealing with—life, at our own humble level and in the best way we could.

So without pursuing those grander options, the optimism we expressed at the time was nothing more than celebrating the moment. We were in between. That in itself was a good place to be, taking a breather, if nothing else. What went before was finally over, successfully finished. What was coming we didn't know, and therefore, in that moment, couldn't hurt. So settling in to a pleasant state of optimism, however temporary, was a pretty good choice.

6

Choose Your Poison

JUDY

I had eight chemo treatments, starting on December 22, 2003, and ending on May 21, 2004. The first four (Adriamycin and Cytoxan, aka AC) were the most difficult in terms of side effects.

I had moments when I absolutely lost it. In fact, the first moment occurred before we had even decided on the chemo regimen. We were scheduled to see the woman who would be our oncologist. The day before our appointment, I got a call from the doctor's office saying that she needed to reschedule our appointment for the following week. Of course, she had a legitimate reason, but I saw only insult and injury. I had been gearing up to the next step, not to waiting. I tempered my response to the person making the call, but I bawled as soon as I hung up the phone. I was outraged and terribly disappointed, and I felt thwarted. I expressed these feelings in my journal: *Everything is testing me, is going wrong, is making me feel worse and worse, causing me to not trust anyone, keeping me focused on negative thoughts, keeping me away from new information and commitment to moving forward …* Dan tried to help me put this glitch into perspective, but to me it stood as something catastrophic.

We finally met with Dr. Caskey, our oncologist, on December 15. We were clearly the newbies in the waiting room—everyone else was more upbeat. I was totally withdrawn, wanting to be invisible. I guess once you get into the routine, you become more comfortable with being there and the veil of mystery of how you will take this treatment is lifted. Clearly you wait a lot both for the treatment and during the treatment, so some form of entertainment is necessary.

Dr. Caskey was very businesslike in reviewing the particulars of my case and in the presentation of the four treatment options, each of which she recommended begin immediately.

A cancer diagnosis is more complex than just a statement that you have "it" in a certain body location. A breast cancer diagnosis also incorporates what kind of cancer it is, how aggressive it is (what grade it is), how big it is and how much it has spread (what stage it is), whether it has hormone receptors, and whether your HER2 (human epidermal growth factor receptor 2) gene is contributing to its growth. That's a lot to deal with, and it takes a while to put all the pieces together. It's information you don't want to deal with in the first place, but it will determine your immediate future.

My breast cancer did not have hormone receptors, meaning it was not triggered or fed by hormones. The majority of breast cancers do have hormone receptors, and therefore, many breast cancer patients take the well-known drug Tamoxifen or its newer relative, Arimidex, two of the available hormone therapies. But since my cancer did not have hormone receptors, taking Tamoxifen would not be part of my treatment protocol. Most people who inquired about my proposed treatments asked if I would take Tamoxifen, because that was a treatment already familiar to them.

The HER2 gene directs cells to produce HER2 growth factor receptors to control the growth and division of cells. Everyone has the HER2 gene, but some patients with breast cancer have a HER2 gene that produces too much of the HER2 protein. Too much HER2 protein makes the cancer grow faster. My HER2 gene was one that "over-expressed" the HER2 protein, so the doctor recommended treatment specific to this condition.

The numbers were laid out on the table. Without any treatment, my chances of recurrence were 60–70 percent—that number startled me. With regular chemo, that chance was reduced by 25 percent. We might be given the option of a clinical trial that would address the HER2 issue, in which case (if we were in the 50 percent that actually got the additional treatment), that number decreased even more. Before the visit to Dr. Caskey, I had not even allowed my mind to consider numbers related to recurrence, or to consider the long-term future at all. "Denial shall make for a better outcome," I was probably thinking. But I'm sure I was expecting much more encouraging news! If I had cancer and I did everything I could to treat it, then it should go away completely and never come back—a child's fairy tale.

DAN

The first visit to the oncologist was a downer.

That's not entirely fair. I suppose we were a little down just being there. The waiting room was a fairly lively place; the upbeat staff was familiar with everyone, exchanging a lot of cheerful banter and good wishes. It was the holiday season, Christmas being only ten days away. But we were newcomers, so there was no familiarity, no joy of recognition, and no positive comparisons to some previous visit. I'm sure everyone was friendly and professional—we simply weren't in the mood for it. We had serious business to attend to. And by choosing to forget that in an oncologist's office *everyone* has serious business to attend to, we felt people should respect the gravity of our situation by keeping their pleasantries to themselves. Of course, when one of the staff offered me a cup of coffee, my mood lightened considerably, though I didn't let on, careful to remain matched to Judy's somber mood.

The doctor herself was a severe person, well suited, I supposed, to the nature of her practice. She was also soft-spoken and serious. Strictly business. Serious business. Over time she showed enough flashes of jolliness to make me reconsider my first impression of her, and looking back I have wondered if she adapted that serious, all-business delivery to match what she thought we needed. That's probably overanalyzing the initial encounter, but I did have difficulty at the time reconciling a dour doctor with the personable and positive staff she had assembled.

Dr. Caskey began by going over the various pathology reports, and while she didn't exactly shake her head and say "tsk, tsk" to indicate how bad it was, that was exactly the impression I received—even without understanding very much of what she described. The delivery, the tone of voice, and the inflection were the clues that things were not at all good. Then she presented some less than encouraging statistics, ones that really shook us up. Basically she told us that an intense round of chemotherapy would only reduce the likelihood of the cancer returning by about one-third. That left Judy with what amounted to a 50 percent chance of recurrence. Needless to say, we were hoping for better odds than that. I wanted to dismiss what Dr. Caskey was saying by ascribing her negativity to what I perceived to be her basic personality. It was only natural, I told myself, that someone so severe would overemphasize the negative. She would guard against optimism, always prepare people for the worst. That's just the way she was. I was trying to convince myself of that, knowing that my efforts were but rehearsal for when I would have to convince Judy of the same thing once we left the consultation.

Going in to that meeting, we were primarily focused on the chemo treatments and getting through them. We had heard they could be devastating, so we were probably geared up to finding out the details of how bad the treatments might be and how best we could get through them. As we saw it, getting through chemo was really all that stood between us and the end of the cancer episode. Neither of us was ready to be told, before we even got to the details of the treatment, that it would be so minimally effective. It became apparent that the consultation was not going as we hoped. Instead of optimism, we were getting yet another helping of bad news, continuing the pattern established after the first two surgeries. These repeated disappointments and negativity were piling up. However correct and realistic Dr. Caskey was being in her assessment, I found myself getting more and more frustrated and primed to vent some of that frustration the next time things didn't go exactly as I expected them to.

Dr. Caskey proceeded to present four treatment options. The first involved two four-dose infusions of different drugs, at intervals of three weeks. A total of eight treatments. The second option was the first option along with participation in a clinical trial. The third option was two four-dose infusions using different drugs from options one and two, also for a total of eight treatments three weeks apart. The fourth option was option three with participation in a clinical trial. Dr. Caskey gave more details as she presented the options, pointing out some specifics of each, then asked for our decision.

That was my cue to act out. "That's not what I want to be doing," I said. "I don't think it is appropriate for us to be choosing from a menu of options. We came here hoping to hear a recommended treatment plan from you, the expert. And if it was something we really didn't like, we would want to hear an alternative recommendation from you, the expert."

Not surprisingly, based on my initial take on her, she responded abruptly, seemingly put out with me. She explained that she had informed us of the differences in the options so that we could make an informed choice. "If something requires more clarification, you only need ask."

"I don't have the background or experience necessary to make an informed decision, and I doubt if I understand enough to even ask a sensible, clarifying question. You are the one with the knowledge and experience. I hardly think this is a situation that calls for participatory decision making. I mean, what if we choose wrong? This isn't the kind of situation where somewhere down the road we have to say, 'Oops, we should have gone with option four instead of one.' Help us out here."

And she did. She prioritized the four options as to what she thought the most appropriate, given the pathology reports. Not surprisingly, we chose the one she put at the top of the list, Option Two. Option Two was four treatments, three weeks apart, of Adriamycin and Cytoxan, what we quickly learned to refer to as AC. The second round would be Taxol, given on the same schedule and for the same duration. The clinical trial was for Herceptin, a drug already used in Canada and Europe and being tested for approval in the United States. It specifically addressed the type of cancer reflected in the pathology reports. Being part of the study did not mean Judy would get the drug; that was a random computer decision. If she was chosen to receive the drug, it would be administered weekly for one year, beginning with the first Taxol treatment. If she was not chosen, she would know that and would not receive a placebo. Chosen or not, she would be required to have regular MUGA (Multi-Gated Blood Pool Scan) tests, a heart monitoring test, as part of the trial.

We met with the clinical trial specialty nurse in Dr. Caskey's office the following day to hear the details of participation. The nurse also went over the anticipated side effects of the AC treatment and explained what countermeasures would be provided and what were available as backup. Dr. Caskey had gone over that with us as well, but hearing it again was a good approach to preparing us. Our follow-up visit also familiarized us with more of the staff, who over the next several months became a new branch of our family.

JUDY

With "quantity" assuming some parameters now, I dove into the quantity vs. quality debate. *I'm not guaranteed any number of days, months, or years, but I am permitted to make the most of each one I get. So perhaps I will most often choose not to use a day in torturing myself on the "why me" and "this is only horrific."* I heard this as a plea and a guiding principle that I either would or would not be able to employ. But the debate brought some comfort and a modest sense of control over my well-being at a time when my life seemed to be falling in on itself.

So even before chemo started, I was feeling raw and highly sensitive, tragic even. *It is absolutely overwhelming what I have to take in ... What an incredible weight I feel! Like nothing I do is working enough, like I have to keep putting out new energy and positivity when I feel so unenergetic and so negative.* This was a very hard mindset, and I felt this way even before I began to feel poorly physically.

Just when I thought things couldn't get any worse, I got my first period in almost a year. Was my entire body falling apart? I was worried that chemo couldn't start until I checked this out. I wrote, *The big boogie tonight is worrying about my gynecological appointment tomorrow—what in hell is she going to tell me? Can I take any more bad news? Do I have a choice? Am I not amazed with myself at taking as much bad news as I already have and still smiling some of the time?*

As this journey became more complicated, I began to realize that I needed to find comfort and hope in something other than the treatment modalities. I needed a visual that would encourage me and remind me of what was important—something I could create and pull energy from. That's how I came to creating my tree of life. It took a while for the image of a tree to come to me, but when it did, it hit me full bore. I would draw a large tree on my big flipchart paper and hang it where it would continually inspire and comfort me. I'm not artistic by any means, but I enjoy cutting and pasting and I felt I could create a satisfying replica of a tree.

My scheme was to name what was feeding me, my roots. The general categories of people, places, and activities seemed to cover what my roots were, but I also added one named "treatment." On the trunk of the tree I hung paper red hearts, on which I wrote the names of those closest to me—family and friends. The branches were numerous and covered with individual leaves, more friends and extended family, some grouped around a shared activity (like book club), others individual.

My tree of life just kept growing, especially as more and more people sent messages—even distant acquaintances. We don't often take the time to identify and appreciate our human riches, but in a crisis it makes so much sense to do just that. When life is going smoothly, we default to taking our fortune for granted; when life is bumpy, we often believe all our fortune is gone. But in reality, it is just one piece of fortune that has changed, and affirming the many pieces of fortune that have not changed gives us a real boost to endure the bumps.

And the kind of tree I chose? Not a standard maple, or oak, or ash—certainly not pine (for how could I fit names on thin needles?). Instead, I picked a gingko tree. I remembered from childhood that the gingko had a unique, fan-shaped leaf that was the most difficult to find for science class leaf collections. In fact, I've rarely seen one outside of my childhood neighborhood in Chicago. When I told my sister Debbie (a gardener) of my choice, she did some research and came back with an article or two on the gingko. I found it affirming to learn that the gingko was the oldest tree in existence; it dated to prehistoric times. Its longevity was credited to its resistance to disease and other blights. This was a tree like what I wanted to be! There was therapy in the physical act of cutting out dozens of leaves and writing names on them (taking a moment with each to think of the person or the experience). And the sum of the parts was amazing. The tree hung in my office for the duration of my treatment—December 2003 through April 2005.

DAN

We were all set to get started. Judy went to the hospital for the baseline MUGA. Then we found out she was chosen to receive the trial drug Herceptin. That was good news. We would have liked to take it as a sign that our luck was changing and that things would start going smoothly, but it didn't happen. Judy—no, Judy's body, which obviously was completely independent of her control—complicated the situation by presenting her with her first period in almost a year. That was a red flag, because while she had not been formally called menopausal, a lapse of more than nine months is usually indicative of menopause. To find out why she was now having a period required an emergency visit to a gynecologist, followed by an ultrasound. The final result of all that extra running around and worrying was that the blood thinner she had been put on was the cause of the bleeding, and, therefore, the bleeding was inconsequential.

In hindsight, I suppose the latest unanticipated bump in the road should have been just one more reminder that nothing was going to be easy in this process. We were unsuspecting participants in yet another clinical trial, one reverifying the efficacy of Murphy's law of things always going wrong. Of course, in the moment, having to deal with the period problem was just one more thing to endure, one more delay in the process. Something that had to be dealt with because there was no choice, something that quickly became unimportant and forgettable as the next event entered and took center stage. In the recounting of the episode it seems like a piling-on penalty should have been called, but in reality, most of the crises simply came, were dealt with, and then went. We had built up not immunity to them, but rather something more akin to a callous. We were hardened. Our skin was thicker, enabling us to absorb the difficulty and work through it without any obvious damage.

We finally reached a point where there was only chemo in front of us. There wasn't time for anything else to go wrong. Our thoughts turned to those we knew who had dealt with chemo, hoping, maybe, to glean one last bit of information or inspiration from the experience of others. Judy's mother underwent two rounds of chemo and never talked about it. Her experience hadn't seemed to be too difficult, though we were a thousand miles away when it was going on and never got to see firsthand. Judy's mother was fairly stoical and fatalistic about those kinds of things. If a treatment was possibly going to help, then any discomfort associated with it was beside the point. She lost her hair, and that was the extent of what any of her children knew about how the chemo was affecting her. Several years earlier, a neighbor of ours, when diagnosed with cancer, refused any treatments. He did not want who he was to be altered by chemicals. He wanted to be himself when he died, which happened fairly quickly. When Judy's friend Gina was undergoing breast cancer treatment a few years earlier, Judy accompanied her to chemo sessions. Gina, however, was determined to be stronger than the chemo and didn't dwell on the details of side effects.

So Judy did not have much to go on as the first treatment drew near. I had even less. And we really didn't talk about it much. I worried when the doctor and the nurse told her what might happen, because, knowing Judy's suggestible side, I suspected that what she was told might happen, *would* happen. This was also probably the only moment during this journey when I wished it were me and not her going through it, simply because I felt that I could endure the treatment better than she could. Of course, that was an easy thing for me to say, not being the one with the chemo port surgically implanted in my chest. I suppose that sort of armchair bravado is as typical as it is pointless. What was the point, however, was imparting to her whatever resources I had that made me so sure I could get through it OK.

If it were me undergoing chemo, I would convince myself that getting through treatment was a matter of time and diversion. Understanding that the chemo side effects would only go on for so long, it would become a matter of focusing my attention on something other than the discomfort. I was not sure Judy would be able to do that. I was hoping to be surprised, but I was not counting on it. I was sure that I would be helping her with just that, trying to distract her as much as I would be holding her hand and reassuring her that she could do it and that the worst would be over soon. It would not be an easy time—I prepared myself for that, having finally learned to ascribe the worst-case-scenario philosophy to everything about this journey. I dreaded the upcoming treatments for how difficult they would be for her, and I also worried how well I could help her. That fear of ineffectiveness and helplessly witnessing her suffering probably prompted my desire to magically trade places with her. Perhaps it wasn't so much that I could do it better; I worried more about being in the "helping" role and failing.

JUDY

My chemotherapy started on December 22. As is our practice, Dan and I had found a synchronicity that gave us support in this new venture. December 22 marks the winter solstice, when the days start getting longer. Diane, a friend who is a medical professional, tried to discourage us from equating chemo with sunshine (because she knew that chemo could have horrific side effects), but we, naively or not, wanted to consider it as something that would heal, that would warm and brighten our days, each day getting better. To support our optimism and also provide comfort, Diane later created a wonderfully symbolic gift of a sun-shaped tote bag that could also serve as a squishy pillow when it was stuffed.

In anticipation of the first treatment, I wrote in my journal, *Today can be called by many names—the last day of waiting, the last day before healing begins, the last day of the known. I'm feeling pretty fragile. And scared about the new stage I'll be entering tomorrow.*

The treatment itself was comfortable. Most of the three hours we were there, we talked with the oncology staff. We went over side effects and red flags to watch for—those were overwhelming! If you dwell on the list, you could make yourself sick just reading it. Common side effects: lowering of white, red, and platelet blood cell counts; nasal irritation; nausea or vomiting; loss of appetite; hair loss; mouth soreness; diarrhea; muscle and joint aching; nerve irritation; numbness and tingling in fingers and toes; allergic reaction; alteration in heart rhythm; changes in skin and nails; and fatigue. Red flags: temperature of 100.5 degrees or higher; chills or other signs of infection; bleeding of nose, gums, or other areas of mouth; bruising without skin trauma; blood in urine or stools; shortness of breath; and painful swallowing.

It didn't hurt that today was sunny. Actually, the chemo room was always sunny, even when the weather was not. The room was made as cheery as possible: comfortable chairs, blankets, pillows, slipper socks, hand warmers, hot chocolate, magazines, books, radio, TV. But best of all were the staff. How did they maintain their calm, their gentleness, their total care and concern? I fell in love with all of them; they held my future in their hands. And they treated it with the utmost care.

The room arrangement lent itself to camaraderie among the patients and caregivers. The nurses were not sealed off in a private room; they were just over the counter, so any time you needed one of them, you only had to speak in a normal voice. And even if you didn't need them, they would check on you continually. I had wondered about how it would feel to be in a room with other patients, and my first instinct was to want to hide out somewhere by myself and distance myself from others. But even though I did not chat a lot with other patients over the course of my treatments, I did feel a sense of community that was comforting. And I learned a lot from them, as they, too, coped with an unwelcome journey.

The second and third days after this particular chemo aren't bad. Steroids are the reason. Then those wear off, and medications intended to relieve side effects cause other complications, like agitation. Within three days of that first treatment, I wrote, *I've been feeling awful. The worst I've ever felt. How can I possibly go through with this?* I couldn't even get myself together enough to share our older son's happiness with the news of an expected grandchild. Chemo had robbed me of my usual positive enthusiasm to such wonderful announcements. Agitation ruled my body and my mind. I felt absorbed with personal details: What did I need to do to feel better? Should I try to eat more? Should I seek more medication? Should I seek distractions? Could I handle much more of this?

My reactions to chemo were profound and multifaceted. I dealt with some nausea, but that didn't seem as bad as I had anticipated. I dealt with bowel irregularities. My white cell count didn't drop until two weeks after the first treatment, but when it did I became feverish and congested and was put on antibiotics. (Fortunately, at no other time during treatment did my white cell count cause me problems, though it stayed on the low side for more than a year after chemo was finished.) I dealt with hair loss (head, eyebrows, eyelashes, nose, and pubic). I dealt with weight loss (that was not an unwelcome side effect). I dealt with loss of taste and increase in smell. I dealt with an alternately congested and drippy nose. I dealt with the knowledge that much of my interior was being negatively affected. I dealt with chemically caused menopause. I dealt with breaking and discolored nails. I dealt with sensitivity to heat. I had what others referred to as "chemo brain," a forgetfulness, fogginess, and general inability to think clearly. And I dealt with depression and anxiety and feeling fragile.

While I despised feeling physically ill, it was the emotional turmoil that hit me harder. I have always been a very positive, upbeat, and optimistic person, and my life has been filled with much happiness. Dan's nickname for me, "Pollyanna," was well earned. Suddenly, I wasn't positive, or upbeat, or optimistic. I had no "go-for-it spirit," even though I was reading and hearing that a go-for-it spirit was what was needed. I continually surprised Dan with a new habit of worrying that certainly was not congruent with being a Pollyanna.

Even as early as my one-week follow-up visit to Dr. Caskey's (after the first chemo treatment) to check my white cell count, I fell apart and surprised Dan with my tears and depression. He thought things had been going well so far. On the ride home, he acknowledged that it would just be that way—up and down—and that's OK. A pattern was establishing itself, at least for the early weeks; I needed to unload occasionally, and then I could move on to more pleasant things.

Some of those pleasant things, however, were not the things I had found pleasant pre-cancer. I had been a longtime listener of a local jazz radio station. But suddenly I felt it was too loud; I didn't want the DJs talking to me any more (as gentle as they were). So for a while I switched to the classical station, and then to CDs. First I listened to CDs on a headset, but when I began to have pangs of loneliness and isolation, I opted for the full-size, room-filling stereo.

Originally I had thought yoga would work for me on my cancer journey. While I did go back to it for a session or two after my surgeries, I no longer found pleasure in doing so. I had been so happy in that yoga environment that I didn't want my current condition and limitations to taint the memory of what it had meant to me before. Yes, I did a lot of deep breathing—that was a real mind saver many times during treatment. But I gave up my practice of yoga postures for almost a year.

Actually, it was difficult for a time to identify pleasant things to do. My world became much smaller for a while. Pleasant meant much less than it had pre-cancer. It now meant the absence of intense discomfort or the ability to feel relaxed rather than tense and frightened, and only that.

DAN

The treatment itself was more of a nonevent than a memory in the making. First they take blood to make sure your blood count is high enough, strong enough, to take the chemo. Since this was Judy's first treatment, there was no concern she would pass. With subsequent treatments it became more of a concern. The treatment drugs target fast-growing cells. They do not discriminate between cancer cells and normal functioning fast-growing cells, which accounts for most of the adverse side effects of the chemotherapy. Blood, hair, and the inside of the mouth, for example, all incorporate fast-growing cells that get "treated" along with the cancer cells. When the chemo destroys red blood cells, the red blood count goes down and there is loss of energy. When the white count drops, the risk of getting sick is heightened. So before the staff can administer the next treatment, they must check the blood count to make sure the levels are high enough to take another hit. If not, the treatment is postponed until the count comes back up. So the blood work was always the first step. Next Dr. Caskey would examine Judy, and, if she passed that test, then she got the infusion.

At the first treatment we met a patient named Millie. Millie was an older woman. Her son, who was about our age, was there with her. Judy was just starting her dose when Millie finished hers. The nurse disconnected the IV, and Millie got up to go to the bathroom a little too quickly, considering she had been sitting for so long. She fell. It was a bad enough fall that an ambulance was called and she was taken to the hospital. We could only hope that this was not a typical day in the chemo room. The nurses, sensing our concern, assured us it wasn't always that eventful. Aside from the trauma associated with finding a vein, for those patients who had not had ports put in, nothing much happened in the chemo room And that was true for Judy. The nurses hooked the tubes up to her port, hung the pouches of chemo on the IV pole, and let them drip. When the bags were empty, they disconnected her, and we went home.

That was December 22. The impact was gradual. On Christmas Eve, our friends Annie and Dave came by to see how Judy was doing. I spoke to them downstairs and then checked with Judy to see if she wanted to see them. She invited them up to the bedroom, and we had a short, cheery visit there. They reminded us we were invited over to their place for their traditional Christmas gathering, but we were pretty sure we would be spending the day quietly at home.

By Christmas day, Judy was effectively knocked out. The only plan we had not cancelled ahead of time was our usual holiday morning walk, but even that never happened. Most of the day she slept, in bed or on the couch. She ate sporadically; not everything tasted good nor tasted consistently. She tried working on a jigsaw puzzle but couldn't summon up the necessary concentration.

Darren came by in the afternoon to visit. Judy was on the couch in the living room at the time, horizontal and under covers. We talked for a while, and then he announced that his partner Alma was pregnant, due in the summer. Normally it is Judy who responds demonstratively to news like that, but she was too wiped out. It took me a moment to realize that the ensuing silence was mine to break. I found the words to express my joy and happiness over the news, but I'm sure part of it sounded as forced as it felt, as if I was trying to salvage the moment. I was, to some extent. I was elated at the news and especially happy for Darren, but the surprise and the contrast with the rest of the day left me rambling awkwardly. I'm sure he had hoped his news would brighten things or maybe even provide a magic elixir for Judy and give her some relief, however temporary. It didn't have that effect, and though she did manage to offer some quiet words of congratulations, she stayed with us only a short while longer before she dragged herself up the stairs to bed. Judy was always enthusiastic, especially regarding a grandchild. Her inability to summon any exuberance over Darren's announcement left us both surprised and worried. Though we didn't speak the words aloud, I think both

Darren and I realized things were happening at a more serious level than we wanted to admit.

She felt better the next day and took advantage by doing things around the house, even going out for a walk. We kept some engagements with friends, but cancelled others, depending on how strong or "right" Judy was feeling. There was no consistency to that. An OK day was usually followed by a day of exhaustion, or if not exhaustion, she was bothered by a bloody nose, or a fever, or constipation, or some symptoms directly related to the chemo.

A week after the first treatment, we returned to the office for a blood test and a let's-see-how-you're-doing visit with Dr. Caskey, I felt fairly optimistic. Sure, there had been some rough moments, but we had also had more than a fair amount of OK-or-better times. Coping with the chemo seemed doable, and I expected Judy to make that brave, optimistic report to the doctor. But when we got into Dr. Caskey's office, Judy exploded into tears and was barely able to relate how terrible and how fragile she felt and how depressed she was. I hadn't seen that coming and probably looked more surprised than the doctor.

And then, only a few minutes later, on the way home, things weren't that bleak. Judy's outburst had managed to quiet the demons for a while.

Our life was beginning to take on a flavor reminiscent of when her father was dying. Like Judy, he was always vibrant and alive, but in his last few months he was reduced to enduring as best he could between doses of painkillers. He would watch the clock, trying to occupy his mind with various activities to make the time go faster. When the time came to take his medicine, he would visibly brighten at the prospect of getting that small measure of temporary relief.

Things were not at that point with Judy, but her life, our life, became centered around dealing with her discomfort. And in addition to the physical discomfort, other problems began to occur. Judy's rapid pulse rate and periods of depression pointed to a growing anxiety. Things were never quite right, or if they were, it was only in short intervals. In fact, nothing—good or bad, physical or emotional—lasted for very long. While half of that was OK, I found it difficult to get a handle on what was going on, let alone come up with an overall approach to help, other than to roll with her current state, wherever that went.

What was coming into focus, slowly, was that chemo was like a new element, a new character entering our lives. It was not readily or easily definable. It was supposed to be a help, yet its presence was so debilitating that we could easily lose sight of its purpose. When people speak of fighting cancer, are they really talking about battling the disease or the treatment? That was no longer clear.

7

Spiraling Down: Searching for a Bottom

JUDY

Chemo was no longer a complete unknown, and so the second treatment didn't have my imagination running quite as wildly. But what I had already discovered about chemo did not make it less frightening. The effects of treatment are cumulative, so on that note, my imagination could still do its dirty work. In that way it was harder to go the second time than the first.

The debilitating side effects of the treatments do subside, and spacing the treatments three weeks apart allows for a brief respite from feeling awful. But other effects start happening. Just before the second treatment, my hair started falling out. *There is hair everywhere. I'm not vacuuming again until it is all out.*

The second treatment was on January 13, 2004, a Tuesday. Again I felt good the next day—thank the steroids for that. We were doing a new anti-nausea protocol—more and better drugs to counteract the chemo drugs. Dealing with treatment is a complex web that involves a lot of trial and error, because each person's reactions are different. The new measures worked for a day or two but proved not to be the right combination.

My crash this time came on Saturday. Fatigue and queasiness were two symptoms I could identify, but they didn't adequately define the "off" feeling that overwhelmed me. I just didn't feel right—like my body was no longer mine but instead was an ill-fitting and hostile costume. I had no control over it. I couldn't generate a familiar response. I couldn't even get it interested in food.

DAN

Her hair started falling out about a week before her second treatment. Just a little each day, but her scalp felt noticeably different to her within a week, though it never got ultrasensitive. Her hair loss could have been more of a shock than it was had I not in previous years seen both Gina and Judy's mother bald, and they both wore that look well. Judy, unfortunately, didn't. It was pretty unsightly, primarily because the hair never completely fell out. There were always a few clumps that resolutely clung to her scalp. I was prepared for the smooth, cue ball look—and even thought I would enjoy rubbing her head for good luck or polishing it with a soft cloth. But instead of the smooth globe, I got the Tolkien orc look, which was a little hard to warm up to. Aesthetically, Judy was also disappointed with the shape and look of her balding pate, so she quickly became proficient with scarves and other manners of headdress. As attractive as she managed to make herself, a scarf wound around a woman's head seemed to announce to the world that she was in chemotherapy and not simply making a fashion statement. It was a calling card.

Also about that time, Judy hooked up with an organization called Qualife. It was amazing how many organizations were out there to provide countless services to cancer patients. (One even gave us tickets to a variety of entertainment events—just gave them to us so we, or anyone in our circumstances, would have a momentary respite from dealing with the disease.) Qualife offered a variety of services, many of which we would utilize later on, but at that moment Judy opted for Reiki therapy. Her first session was pleasant, and a nice diversion, but it seemed to have no lasting benefits. That's not a reflection on Reiki or the therapist, that's just the way things were then with Judy. Nothing was extremely good, and what was even marginally good didn't hang around very long.

From my perspective, there were enough OK days in a row and she was doing enough normal activities that I had no visible indication she was overly concerned about going to the second treatment. Of course, based on her explosion at Dr. Caskey's office a week after the first treatment, I was not very confident in my ability to read her. More likely, I probably convinced myself that the impact of the first chemo treatment really wasn't all that bad. I guess I wanted to believe that, just as I wanted to believe that subsequent sessions would be easier, since we knew what to expect. The truth was—and I am not sure when in the process I first heard these warnings, or when the import of them finally sank in—each treatment of chemo can produce different side effects, and the effects are cumulative. Not yet grasping all that probably helped me help her get to the second treatment.

The treatment went without the drama of the first one, and for the first three days nothing seemed to be amiss. During that time we attended the funeral of our friend Mary's mother. The funeral service was on the east side of town, and the cemetery was on the extreme west edge. When Judy assured me she felt well enough to drive, I agreed, appreciating the opportunity to leave the driving to her. Except that her driving totally unnerved me. Her reflexes seemed slow. I guessed it might have been all the additional anti-side effect medication she was taking after the treatment, but once we agreed that she would drive, I didn't want to insist that she wasn't sharp enough. So it was a nerve-racking ride across town, twice, mostly to do with her judgment of braking distance. Rear-ending someone while in a funeral procession seemed a particularly uncool thing to do, but she was confident she was up to the task. I managed to confine the expression of my concern and criticism to unsubtle body language, most notably slamming both feet into an imaginary brake pedal on the passenger side while I thrust my arms into the dashboard to brace myself for the coming impact.

On the third day after chemo, a Friday, she began to feel a little fatigued, and by Saturday she felt what she could only describe as "off." She was no more communicative than that. No details. Just "off." And with no visual or physical symptoms to accompany that one verbal complaint, I had nothing specific to address. I could only stand by, keep up the routine, and hope that "off" would prove to be both a mild and short-lived side effect. But that night, while sitting at the dinner table and not eating her dinner, she broke the quiet by softly announcing, "If I ever have to go through this again, I won't."

I was stunned. There was defeat in her voice as well as her words. While I had expected a variety of situations, I doubt I ever gave much thought to one in which Judy gave up. That was just so unlike her, and certainly not a scenario I wanted to consider and prepare for, because frankly it was the one I felt least competent dealing with. But there it was, right across the table from me. I went around to her and put my arms around her. "I won't hold you to that," I whispered. We held on to each for a while, and then she went to bed.

JUDY

Dan had a rough day yesterday watching me be so miserable. When I said I didn't think I could go through with this, he persuaded me to consider the alternative and to believe that I did have the ability to go through with it. He would change places with me if he could. He doesn't want to see me go through this. I'm really a wimp about pain and when I'm feeling pain, I can't imagine living through it. My sense of proportion of the importance of things gets all screwed up when I'm hurting. I feel like I don't want to be around because I hurt so bad, and I don't have any thoughts about what I would miss if I weren't around, what others would miss if I weren't around, etc. It's totally fragmented, and I'm seeking immediate relief.

By Sunday I couldn't handle it on my own anymore. I called one of the oncology nurses at her home, a number she had generously offered. At my first call (11:00 AM), she suggested taking an additional anti-nausea pill to pick me up. At my second call (4:30 PM), she suggested a different anti-nausea pill. At my third call (6:30 PM), she suggested I come to the office in the morning for IV fluids. Most of the day I'd lain around, unable to fall asleep. I was agitated and uncomfortable and worried. I could not describe to Dan what I needed other than to talk to medical professionals, and that was not producing any lasting result. My assumption was that if they were putting their drugs into me, they should know what I needed to enable me to tolerate them. I was expecting an exact science, but wasn't getting it.

Mentally I was a mess. *Whiny, totally lethargic, negative, depressed, unable to muster any positive attitude ...* I was in a spiral, and I could not help myself. After my third call to the oncology nurse failed to bring any immediate relief, I went higher and phoned the on-call doctor. My hysteria convinced him that I needed to go to the hospital for IV fluids. I didn't know exactly what IV fluids I needed, having latched onto that idea from the nurse I had just spoken to, but I assured him I wouldn't make it through the night without immediate help. Within an hour Dan and I were at the hospital, and I was admitted to the Infusion Center. The doctor had prepared the staff for my arrival and had ordered a three-hour IV dose for me, a combination of anti-anxiety medication, anti-nausea medication, and basic IV fluids (potassium chloride). The comfort of the hospital was real for me; I felt better just being taken care of. When we got back home late that night, I easily fell asleep, and by the next morning I felt good.

DAN

A Sunday morning in mid-January normally would find me settling into a day full of football playoff viewing. Judy was weak, in addition to still feeling off, so it looked like she would spend most of the day in bed, which freed me to vegetate in front of the television, trusting that my batteries would get a chance to recharge during the rest. We assumed our positions, and the day started off as planned.

Just before noon, I heard her talking to someone on the phone. The phone had not rung, so she must have called someone. By listening to what she was saying, I determined she had called the nurse from Dr. Caskey's office who had given Judy her home number in case she needed help getting through the weekend. Judy explained what was wrong, emphasizing her queasiness and overwhelming anxiousness. The nurse calmed her and recommended that she take more of one of the medications. That worked for a while, but later in the afternoon she was on the phone with the nurse again. "Something's going wrong," Judy insisted. "This is more than just side effects." The nurse recommended she take something else.

Judy did not involve me in this process. She made the first call when I thought she was sleeping. Afterward, she told me what the nurse had recommended, then she took the medication and returned to bed. Again I thought she was sleeping when I heard her on the phone the second time. I was unsure what to do. I felt that at the least I should make the calls for her, but it was apparent she needed to establish direct contact. Rather than filtering through me the information about how she felt, she needed to be sure the nurse understood what was wrong and heard how desperate she was. It was probably the best way to handle the situation. I doubt I would have been able to convey Judy's needs as effectively, because I am not sure I understood them. I was not ready to buy into Judy's theory that it was something other than side effects, but at the time, like Judy, I needed to defer to the health care professionals. And since they were dealing with her calls, and not writing her off as overreacting, I would do the same. Had I been the one making the calls for her, I probably would have been asked to ascertain how much of Judy's problem was emotional and mental, rather than physical. Was she just being a hypochondriac? Did she really have such a low tolerance for pain and discomfort? And then I would likely be asked to try to calm her down and help her through the really rough times. I wasn't ready to step into that role without knowing for sure that there really wasn't something more going on. I guess I needed assurance as well as Judy did, so her bugging the nurse at home on a Sunday seemed the best strategy to achieve the certainty we both needed.

At dinnertime, Judy called the nurse a third time. The nurse was out of ideas and could only suggest that Judy somehow get through the night and come to the office the next day. Apparently that was not good enough for Judy, because she quickly got back on the phone and called Dr. Caskey. She reached the on-call doctor who was covering for Dr. Caskey and convinced him she believed she was dying. The doctor called the hospital and arranged for Judy to be given an IV treatment to provide hydration and sedation. It was a three-hour treatment, and it seemed to do the trick. Judy was a different person when we left late that Sunday night—relaxed and positive. That feeling lasted through the next day. She ate well, making up for a couple of days of barely eating. She even woke early to take me to work so she could have the car all day. She had a Reiki appointment at Qualife and then an appointment to order a wig.

JUDY

That Monday I wrote, *It is so bad when it's bad, and now today I feel so much better!* I was tempted to conclude that it had just been a bad thirty-six hours, but I wasn't comfortable with that. I felt different than I had after the first chemo treatment, and I wasn't confident that when I woke, even after the hospital visit, I would feel better. I worried what the bottom was going to be. And the concern was legitimate, because events proved there was still a lot of down below me.

Several days later, I wrote, *It was really a hell of a week … I lost control many times, and it wore me out and made me more depressed than I already was.* The hospital trip on Sunday night had been followed by a trip to the doctor on Tuesday for more fluids. I thought I felt better but soon freaked out again. Over the phone with an oncology nurse I worked hard to concentrate on deep breathing and kept that up for twelve hours, an amazing concentration of will. Sometimes I could get myself very calm, but then my anxiety would start all over again. It was vicious. I felt out of control.

Dan was completely stressed over the unpredictability of my well-being. He wanted to help. But when I was down, I dragged him down with me. I believe the effects of the second chemo treatment were confusing, both physically and emotionally. And I think at this time I was first aware that my thinking processes were being compromised. I agreed with Dan that we didn't know all we needed to about side effects and that we would continue to ask questions and talk about what was happening. But I knew he was seeking clearer answers than might be possible. Because the effects were happening to me, and not to him, my ideas were being influenced by how I felt; since how I felt kept changing, my ideas kept changing. It was very stressful to impact someone else's life like that. And I needed him so much at that time.

Emotional side effects were not the only problems. I was also bothered by physical side effects, including mouth sores and headaches, along with taste buds and smell buds that produced unappealing sensations. There wasn't a part of me that felt whole any longer.

This marked the time when I started reducing my activities. I gave up my storytelling; I decided I didn't want the students to witness the changes I was undergoing. I previously enjoyed Feldenkrais and massage sessions but no longer felt I could afford the additional expense. Plus my massage therapist expressed concern about continuing my massages: she worried that massage might somehow be bad for me. (I had previously heard this concern from my friend Cathlin. Several years earlier, with her own diagnosis, she had been unable to find a therapist to give her massages. Fortunately I would soon find a welcoming massage therapist through Qualife, but in the early treatment phase I did without. Happily, massage therapists are now enlightened about the benefits of body therapies for people with cancer.)

My current life seemed to want to separate from my previous life. I had been working with a personal coach for six years, but it seemed beside the point under the circumstances. Dan and I even gave up going to movies (from diagnosis to July 2004), because I was ultrasensitive about content and surprises, as well as not very comfortable out in public. Finally, I gave up my responsibilities as editor of a newsletter just to relieve myself of a task I didn't feel up to doing.

Many of these activities were ones I had thought might help me through the worst of chemo by getting me to focus on something else. They were things I was comfortable and familiar with and which had always provided me with pleasure and a sense of fulfillment. But they had lost their appeal, their magic. Having to continue with them seemed burdensome—more to endure, when I was already enduring so much. And, whether I realized it at the time or not, when I gave them up I was giving myself over to whatever the cancer and the chemo had in store for me. I was no longer even pretending to be in charge.

All along I was reading books about cancer and other people's experiences with it. I would read some and then take a break so I wouldn't overwhelm myself, so I wouldn't focus solely on the topic of cancer. Often my readings were helpful, but sometimes they were not, especially when they talked about cancer as being life-changing. That really goes without saying. But here I was, believing that I had a wonderful life; I was already doing what I really wanted to. And the books were saying that I needed to make changes in order to live a more wonderful life! I understand that books like that have to take a hopeful and encouraging tack, but this expectation was burdensome. I resented the pressure to make the improvements I felt the authors exhorted, and I worried that if I didn't make improvements I wasn't "doing it right."

DAN

The following day, Tuesday, I went to work early as usual. It proved to be a busy day. I buried myself in my work as soon as I arrived and thought of nothing else until my shift was over. Judy had not crossed my mind until I was on my way home. Since I received no call from home, I presumed Judy's rebound had carried over, and I hoped we might be through the worst of the second treatment. But no news is not always good news. When I got home, I learned that Judy had had a rough and busy day. Feeling tentative and nervous and experiencing some hot flashes, she had taken a taxi to Dr. Caskey's office to get some more of the IV treatment that had worked so well on Sunday night. Except this time it did not prove as effective. While I was trying to simultaneously digest everything Judy was telling me and deal with my impact to this latest disappointment, Judy was back on the phone with Dr. Caskey's nurse. Just two hours after the latest IV treatment, Judy was already feeling physically devastated. Her anxiety was overwhelming her, and I was starting to feel the same way.

It was becoming obvious to me that without the direct contact of a health care professional, Judy was not going to feel safe. What was happening to her body was so foreign to her, so off, so wrong, she could not accept that it could be a side effect of the treatment designed to rid her body of cancer. Something with that noble a mission should not be creating the devastation her body was experiencing. It was incongruous. Something must have gone wrong, and only the medical community could figure out what. So she reached out to them and insisted they do something to save her. Cancer could kill her. That she understood. Being treated for cancer should not kill her, yet she felt it was. Something had to be done. And that something could not be done by an ordinary person like me. I could offer comfort and help through some crises, but I had no long-lasting magic. I had to turn her over to those who did. Doctors for sure. Better still would be a stay in the hospital until they got everything fixed up right. She needed to be taken care of by the experts.

As a rule, I don't like feeling inadequate. I like to think that I am a pretty capable individual and that I can pretty much do anything I set out to accomplish. Of course, I can only hold on to that belief when what is to be accomplished is something I have control over. Trying to get someone else to change her mindset is not one of those things. It was becoming apparent that Judy needed more than I could give her. Comfort and support and assurances and always being at her side were not enough to quell the demons that had taken her over. That became painfully apparent when she didn't call me that Tuesday to take her to the doctor. I was bypassed by the immediacy of her need. Calling a taxi would get her closer to what she needed faster, and that was what was motivating her then. To some extent that may have been a hard thing to accept, but given the situation, I probably thought it was a good sign that she still had the drive and the energy to go out and get what she wanted. I was always looking for the best spin, which I suppose is an indication of unacknowledged desperation.

That she might be going a little nuts didn't really enter into my thinking. That she might be overreacting to and exaggerating the side effects did occur to me. Such behavior was not a foreign element to her personality. Or mine, for that matter. For one of our anniversaries, I gave Judy a writing journal in which I had headed several of the blank pages with a sentence relevant to our lives together. One message was, "We make mountains out of molehills because mountains are special." The meaning I was conveying there was that we tended to celebrate the little things, like inflating the importance of a shared meal, a walk in the park, or a really funny movie into something heroic, even magical. It was a nice, positive sentiment, but in watching Judy respond to the chemo, I began to see its other edge. Yes, we did accentuate the positive, but accentuating can be habit forming, and pretty soon it might be the negatives that are getting blown out of proportion.

I had to weigh that as I struggled with how best to help her during the worst moments. But while that tendency of ours may have been a contributing factor, what Judy was going through was primarily the result of her mind and body being suddenly inundated with strange and strong new drugs. That entitled her to a fair amount of slack, something which Dr. Caskey's staff and the hospital considered when they repeatedly accepted her need for medical services. They did not question her toughness, her personality quirks, or her sanity. They listened to her symptoms and took steps to restore her to a state of comfort. They didn't suggest she was imagining the symptoms. They didn't suggest she should "toughen up" and "take it like a man." And because they were continuing to deal with her in a straightforward way, I would as well. I could think to myself that she needed a different kind of help, that she didn't need to be indulged so unconditionally by everybody, that in the long run it was not doing her any good. But that was the point: there was no long run. The chemo effects were not forever. They would dissipate, and the key thing was just getting through them. So if Judy needed an inordinate amount of help and attention to get through them, then, absolutely, that was what she should get. It was not the time to be retooling her psyche. If going a little nuts helped get her through this, then that was as good a reason as any. And if we needed to have a doctor or nurse hold her hand or give her a dose of something every day to get her through, we would, as long as *they* would.

8

It's Not Just Physical

JUDY

Dr. Caskey and her team were successfully managing my physical issues, but when I began having panic attacks, she knew I needed additional support. I wrote in my journal, *I have a lot of tears to shed. I have a lot of attitude adjustment to work on so that I don't stay in this scared, shut-down mode all the time. Even when I feel OK, I'm nervous about how long it will actually last.*

By 4:30 AM Wednesday, January 21, I couldn't keep it together any longer, and after crying to Dan for nearly an hour, I called Dr. Caskey. I seemed to have reached a wall; I couldn't soothe myself. The doctor attempted to assure me that my reactions were more emotional than physical and suggested I go to the ER for a mental health evaluation. I wasn't offended at the suggestion; in my need, it was another helping hand—a professional opinion that was credible to me.

DAN

It's not unusual for me to wake up in the middle of the night. The alarm goes off at 4:00 AM, and that is pretty much the middle of the night. If my internal clock stirs me a little before, it is not a problem. I use the extra time to orient myself. I remember what day it is and what I have to gear up for. The extra few minutes of sleep are never as valuable as spending the time convincing myself I have something worthwhile to get up and do. Even at four in the morning.

It was Wednesday. Usually I am off on Wednesdays, but I had been cross-training with another job at work, and Wednesday is a big day for that other position. I couldn't complain about the extra hours and the extra expectations; my employer had been pretty flexible and supportive when I needed to be off with Judy. This was just a little payback—unspoken, un-demanded, but compelling for me just the same.

I was fully awake and decided to turn over to see exactly what time it was. It was only 3:45, but my movements alerted Judy that I was awake.

"You can't go," she said to me.

I wasn't as awake as I thought, at least not to the point that I fully comprehended what she said. "Of course I have to go. They're expecting me. Remember?"

"You can't go," she repeated. "You can't leave me alone."

She cried, and I tried to comfort her, to get her calmed down enough that I could consider going to work. Nothing seemed to work, and her tears kept coming. Judy was not by nature a crier, though she was not hard-core about never crying. It was just that for most of the time I had known her, some forty years, crying was never typical. There were occasions, of course, isolated incidents. When she did cry, it was minimal and therapeutic, as when her parents died. There had been no great wailing episodes like she was having that morning. In the past, mostly I would associate her crying with moments of extreme frustration and anger, usually relating to me or one of the boys when nothing she did seemed to have any impact on us. I suppose her tears that morning were similarly evoked. She must have been frustrated and angry that things weren't going well, and maybe additionally afraid for what that might mean. Whatever the reason, the episode lasted a long time, only ending when she abruptly got out of bed.

I wasn't sure what to do at that point. It crossed my mind that perhaps it was time for a little tough love. It wasn't so much that I was concerned about missing more time at work as I was about helping Judy turn the corner on this. She shouldn't be giving in to this as readily as she was. I felt a little more secure in asking her to rise above the discomfort, because I was fairly certain nothing out of the ordinary was going on, at least in a physical sense. She had been with enough doctors and nurses over the past three days to confirm that. So I determined that it was as good a time as any to broach how well she was handling this. Except that as I was formulating exactly how I would put that determination into words, Judy was back in bed talking to someone on the phone.

Not surprisingly, it was Dr. Caskey she had called. What surprised me was that Judy had gotten through to her so quickly. I sat up and listened to Judy's half of the dialogue. It soon became clear that Judy was repeating everything Dr. Caskey was saying so I could hear both sides of the conversation. "It's not a physical problem," Judy repeated. Then after listening for a while, "You think I should go to the emergency room and get a mental health evaluation. Right away."

There was no argument or defensiveness in Judy's voice. She did not try to convince the doctor that she wasn't crazy, that the discomfort was real and more intense than she could handle. On the other hand, there was no defeat or resignation in her voice as she accepted the doctor's orders. But it was not a passive acquiescence. It was more akin to having just consulted a specialist on a perplexing problem and agreeing this was the next logical thing to try. Judy even seemed optimistic that this might work, and because it might, she was eager to get going.

JUDY

Another ride to the hospital brought relief. Once I was given some Ativan, I calmed down enough to talk with a mental health specialist, who recommended that I pursue a therapeutic path. He gave us a list of names of some individual therapists.

Here's where our story takes a lovely and rewarding twist. On the list was the name of someone Dan knew. It was comforting to be able to start our search with a known quantity, even though Dan believed she would refer us on because of her familiarity with us. He reached her immediately and filled her in. She informed him that she indeed was the right person for me, and we set an office visit for two days hence.

Amazingly, I was able to socialize that night. Was it the Ativan? Was it knowing I would soon be getting additional help? The roller coaster doesn't let you know why it changes direction.

But the next day the panic attacks came again, and even though Dan helped me regain some calm, I remained nervous about when they would recur.

DAN

Dr. Caskey had called ahead to the hospital, so we got ushered right to a bed in the ER. The nurses started an IV, again probably on Dr. Caskey's orders. They pulled the curtain, and there we waited for an awfully long time. The only other patient in the area was a man just coming out of an alcoholic stupor. He was very insistent on being released so he could go to work, a request that the staff found somewhat amusing and predictable. They kept assuring him he was not going anywhere, and he kept insisting his presence there was just a mistake, a misunderstanding. When he finally decided that silence might better serve his case, a group consisting of one ER staff, a security person, and what I gathered was an ambulance driver, filled the silence with reminiscences of some of their most humorous and bizarre late-night, real-life ER episodes. They were having a good time swapping stories, though I was a bit perturbed having to listen to them. It was bad enough to wait so long, but having to hear anecdotes that accelerated in crudeness and graphic detail focused in me some pent-up anger and frustration that I wasn't aware was so close to the surface. At one point I jumped up and said, "That's about enough of that," but to my surprise Judy wondered what I was talking about. She hadn't noticed the chatting. The safeness of being in the hospital, and the IV doing its miracle work, had rendered her pretty much oblivious to the conversations that were so irritating to me. My point became moot, as the brief exchange between us must have reminded the staff they were not alone, and the group broke up.

When the social worker arrived, we moved into a small room, where he asked a bunch of introductory, background questions. Then, ready to get into the heavier, perhaps more delicate stuff, he tactfully asked Judy if she wanted me to leave the room while they talked. I wasn't ready for that but immediately understood it for the practical protocol it was. I was ready for whatever response she gave. It had never occurred to me that I might be part of her problem, but at that point finding out would have been enough of a relief to counteract any hurt I might have experienced. Continuing as the past few days had unfolded was not an option. "Oh, no," Judy said. "We have no secrets. And I need him here to fill in the parts I'm not going to remember all that clearly."

The man nodded his agreement, but I still sensed some suspicion on his part. I found it very satisfying to be held under suspicion. Maybe I needed attention and didn't realize it and—like so many who feel ignored—was willing to accept even negative attention if that was all that was being offered. I would have liked to wallow in my paranoia a while longer, but the interview was proceeding and required my input. In the end, it became apparent that there were no complex and intricate psychological issues at work in Judy's case. It was this simple: she was afraid the chemotherapy was killing her, and no assurances from anybody could convince her otherwise. She wasn't supposed to feel as bad as she did, ever.

After the interview, we returned to our curtained cubby in the ER and waited. When the social worker joined us, he reiterated that the regimen of chemicals Judy was getting was creating sensations and a reality totally unfamiliar to her. It was hard to know what was real, what was more serious than an anticipated side effect of the chemo. Not knowing, not being sure of your own body was a frightening situation. He indicated that getting into regular counseling or therapy was appropriate to help Judy deal with the fear she was experiencing.

We had not opted for that kind of assistance early on in the diagnosis. In hindsight that may have been foolish, even reckless. But before we signed up to do penance for our error, we only had to remember that it had been a small tumor that was detected early. We had thought the whole process would only be a damn inconvenience. All the surgeries were manageable. All the people we knew who had chemo handled it OK, and they were our only role models. And, also in our defense, so many things happened so fast that there was not much opportunity to revisit our knee-jerk, instinctive decision that we could do it all without any outside assistance. The early-morning trek to the ER for a mental health evaluation provided reason and opportunity to revisit the issue, and at that point the decision was an easy one to make. The question was more of whom to see, and for that the social worker presented us with a list of therapists he felt comfortable recommending.

While they were removing Judy's IV in preparation for us going home, I read through the list. Of the four or five names printed there, one struck me as familiar. It was someone I knew, but the first name was different.

"I know her," I said. "I know her as Scotty, but the name on her office is Sharon." And that's how the social worker had listed her. I then went on to remind Judy that Scotty had led a writing workshop I had taken just a few months earlier. The workshop was about committing oneself to writing, and one of the participants had complained it was more like group therapy than a writing workshop. Well, it was like therapy because Scotty was a therapist, and committing oneself to writing involved getting past some psychological and behavioral blocks. But I had always associated Scotty with writing, and when the idea of finding a therapist came up, I doubt if I would have thought of her on my own. So if the visit to the ER room that morning did nothing else, it got Scotty involved.

According to Judy's journal, we went for a walk after we left the hospital that morning. I don't remember that. It would have made more sense that we went out to breakfast, as I must have been starving by that time. In any event, we didn't immediately go home but instead spent some time talking about the next step. I told her I didn't believe Scotty would agree to be her therapist because of the familiarity she already had with me. Still, I felt I could rely on her to recommend someone to us, off our list or from her own experience.

When we got home I immediately called her. I first asked about her daughter, who, I remembered from the workshop, was expecting a baby. Scotty said she was due any moment and that she had hoped my call was the one telling her it was time. I apologized for being the wrong caller and then went on to explain the situation with Judy and told her that we would appreciate a recommendation. "Oh, no," she said. "I'm the one for the job."

I suppose that by that time in the experience nothing should have surprised me, but there I was again—completely floored. That was not at all what I was expecting to hear. She rescued me from my ensuing stuttering and stumbling by saying, "She'll need someone close to her in age. More experienced. No, I'm the one. But just to be proper about it, read me the other names on your list." I did, and she responded with a "good, but too young" or "you don't want a man for this" or a straightforward "don't know her or him."

Judy was watching me as I talked and listening to the tone of my voice. She saw and heard enough. When I was concluding my conversation by telling Scotty I would have Judy call her, Judy reached for the phone and said she'd talk to her right then. I left them talking as I belatedly went to work, much relieved.

When I came home later that afternoon, Judy informed me she had set an appointment with Scotty for Friday. She also told me she was feeling well enough to go dancing that night. And she felt good enough to keep the arrangements to have our grandson over the next day. I would be off work as well, so just in case her sudden rebound didn't last, I was there to cover for her.

JUDY

I haven't talked with any other cancer patient or survivor who doesn't mention the roller-coaster effect of treatment. And yet each of us is taken by surprise when the effect hits us, no matter how many times it hits. When you feel good you can't imagine feeling poorly, and when you feel poorly you can't imagine feeling good. But then something happens (medication side effects or lack of medication side effects), and the feeling changes. That's the bad and the good, I guess. We all can perk up with support and our own inner guidance, but that doesn't prevent downturns—and we learn that lesson repeatedly on this journey.

When Scotty, my new therapist, called the next afternoon to say that she would have to reschedule because her daughter was in labor, I broke down and pleaded with her to stop at our house first. She agreed. I'm so very grateful she did, and so apologetic at the same time, because as a result she missed being present at the birth of her second grandchild. Instead, she came to our house and visited with me until I was calmer and more confident that I could survive my intense anxiety. We scheduled a session for the following week, not in her office, but in our home. This was the pattern that we followed for many months. Scotty was a tremendous resource. She came to know me quickly within my own surroundings, and I was much relieved not to have to pack up my concerns and bring them into a less comfortable setting. I think meeting in a client's home has many wonderful benefits, and I was very grateful for this option.

Scotty helped us look to other resources, first off my sister Laurie, a nurse. I was afraid of being alone and knew I would appreciate having someone around all the time. Dan had been shouldering that responsibility up to now, but he needed some relief, whether he admitted it or not. So we called Laurie, and she made plans to come from Chicago as soon as possible.

Scotty and I started with frequent therapy sessions, and I used Ativan on a regular basis for a while. Medication helped me get through the roughest emotional times. I also started taking an antidepressant. It was a relief to realize that something could ease part of the suffering. Of course, it would take up to six weeks for the antidepressant to achieve its intended effects, but something psychological must have tided me over during that wait time. I was grateful for the calming of my mind, and I was grateful to feel more capable in dealing with day-to-day and long-term issues.

DAN

As it turned out, her rebound did not last. Late Thursday morning Judy had what can only be called a panic attack. Physically something started to bother her and when the discomfort increased to the point where she couldn't concentrate on being with Spencer, she started to worry. She didn't put the worries into words, so I could only imagine what she was afraid of—that she wouldn't get better, that she would not be able to spend time with Spencer, that the cancer would get her as it did her parents and her grandmother. Once she started to think that way, she was less and less in control of herself, and less and less responsive to me or anyone else. She did manage to calm down that day, but not for long. She grew more and more anxious as the day wore on. In the midst of that decline, Scotty called to say her daughter was in labor and to prepare Judy for the possibility of changing Friday's appointment. I don't think Scotty was yet aware of the extent of the problem that prompted the appointment in the first place. She experienced it right at that moment, however, when Judy asked her, and then pleaded with her, and finally convinced her, to come over to the house immediately.

On the way, she picked up some lemon drops, to help quell the chemo nausea, in case we didn't have any in the house. Judy and Scotty then went off to another room to do some breathing exercises and guided imagery, while I amused Spencer until Alex picked him up. I then waited. When Judy was calm again, the three of us talked.

Scotty chaired the meeting. The first thing she suggested was for Judy to start taking her anti-anxiety medicine regularly, not just as needed. I was surprised to learn that she was not taking it routinely. It seemed such a simple and obvious step to take, yet for some reason Judy used the medication sparingly, even though she was taking well below the maximum allowed daily dosage. Somewhere along the line she had gotten into a minimalist mentality when it came to taking medicine. "As needed" meant rarely, if ever—show 'em how tough you are by using so much less than they prescribe. And while that may have been laudable in some circumstances, it was not the appropriate approach for the situation we were in.

The second thing we talked about was getting someone to come and stay with Judy, to help her combat the fear that seemed to intensify whenever she was alone. Judy's sister Laurie was the first and obvious choice. The fact that Laurie was a nurse was a big factor, and the fact that she was good company made it another one of those oh-so-obvious solutions that we couldn't believe we hadn't thought of sooner.

The third thing we talked about was prompted by a phone call Scotty received while she was still at the house. The baby had been born. Her second granddaughter.

Our approach was changing. In retrospect, that Wednesday—certainly that entire week beginning with the calls to Dr. Caskey's nurse—was the turning point in the ordeal. It was the bottoming-out point, even though there were enough difficult days ahead that we couldn't see that clearly at the time. Every difficult day seemed like a new bottom when it was happening, but the ones that came later had more of a temporary feel to them. They were not so fraught with bleakness; they didn't seem as deep and desperate. Things seemed more doable, less fragile. Judy became more open to suggestions.

Our friend Mary came on Saturday to be with Judy while I went to work. They made a batch of ginger snaps. There were no panic attacks that day. Whether that was due to the company or the medication regimen was not important. Something was working.

Laurie arrived the next day, Sunday, January 25, 2004. It was our thirty-fourth wedding anniversary. There was some irony in that, some symmetry. Our actual wedding day had also been a Sunday. We were married at Judy's parents'

home. One of our favorite pictures from that day is one of Judy and Laurie sharing a heartfelt moment. Our marriage represented the first permanent dispersing
of their family unit, the point when life was never going to be the same for anyone. In the picture Judy seems to be comforting her tearful sister. Thirty-four
years later, Laurie arrived to do the same.

9

Calling Out the Cavalry

JUDY

If you don't experience your emotional response in the moment, you will experience it at some future time. At some point along the way, Dr. Caskey informed me that patients who completely fall apart are more likely to rebuild their lives better once they are through the rough treatment times. Did she say that just to give me validation and encouragement, or was it truly her experience? When I heard this statement from others, also, I realized it was not just one of comfort.

Falling apart was what I needed to do for myself, but it was hard on others, at least initially. Maybe it was hard on them until I did successfully rebuild. I was unpredictable, and that is always difficult for others to deal with. I wasn't my usually positive and engaged self. I was showing a different side, a new me that was a creation of the experience. I needed to be authentic to that creation. I couldn't be Judy-as-usual.

I thought about my parents and how they had handled their cancer journeys. When my father was dying from lung cancer in 1978, a team of hospice caregivers visited the house one day, and as a family we sat around the table discussing what my father could do with his time. I remember being engaged in the conversation and really wanting to be the one to suggest something that would make him happier, that would pass the time better. I got it in my head to suggest working with family photographs, sorting and labeling them so our history would be documented better. Now, if someone had suggested that to me when I was feeling poorly, I'm sure I would have had a reaction similar to my father's. He put out a weak and brief effort. It wasn't something that he wanted to do. And being who I was at the time, I probably took it personally that he hadn't embraced my suggestion.

When my mother was dying from ovarian cancer in 1997, I was still giving advice. (Just as people would give me advice during my cancer journey.) I thought my mother "should be" more emotional, more talkative during her last days. In hindsight, with my own experience teaching me differently, I believe other people's perspectives and advice are only good for themselves. I truly cared about my mother and father, but I wasn't walking in their shoes. When I recommended what I thought they should be doing, I really wanted them to do something for me—one more thing for their daughter. Maybe I thought that keeping them occupied with their parental roles would help them hang on longer. It was a form of denial on my part, as well as a failure to grasp what they were really going through. I later came to accept that both of them did the best they could with what they knew at the time—just as I would do years later. And each of us chose a different way. My father stayed angry until his death; my mother stayed reticent. I was emotional and verbal and a mess before I was able to rebuild my world. There are no "should do's" in how you experience your cancer or any other catastrophe. Rather, it is time to go inside and find out how you need to experience it.

And when I went inside myself, even with the adjusted medication and the addition of therapy, I found myself feeling terribly lonely. I didn't want Dan to go to work, and I wanted to see the rest of the family more. I needed to share with others this lost feeling. Part of my relapse into negativity came right after Laurie's visit ended. She had stayed for ten days. Her nursing experience was a great comfort to me. *It is good for me to have someone who can handle the medical details and offer comfort in understanding them and encouragement about trusting the professionals.* But I also wrote, *I am nervous about the third chemo treatment, and I am nervous about Laurie leaving.*

DAN

Sometimes when the cavalry comes, the day is won, the movie ends, and everyone lives happily ever after. On other occasions, the cavalry rides into a trap and the would-be rescuers need rescuing themselves. And every so often the cavalry's very presence so alters the landscape that the original crisis magically fades into the background, making the rescuers superfluous—in which case the cavalry returns to the fort, thus creating a void that the crisis quickly fills up. That's probably not an easy metaphor to follow, but trust me, it works perfectly. Especially the last part of it.

Laurie arrived two weeks after the second AC treatment and just a couple days after the week-long anxiety crisis that had prompted the first call for reinforcements. Just calling her had had a calming effect. The addition of Scotty, and then Laurie, to the on-hand support team brought a certain amount of relief to me and I assumed would have an even more profound effect on Judy. On Monday, the day after Laurie arrived, I went to work more relaxed and more certain that I could lose myself in my work without worrying about being called home immediately. And while I didn't get called away from work, neither did I come home to the positive, upbeat circumstances I anticipated.

Judy and Laurie had spent the day together, primarily catching up. They had also gone to a class for cancer patients on how to apply makeup. Now, I did not recall any warnings that Judy might lose her ability to understand the concept of cosmetics just because she had cancer. I understood that the class was simply an excuse for an outing and an activity. Since Judy had never been heavily into makeup, I assume she approached it from that perspective: it might just be something fun to do. Unfortunately, she wasn't feeling well enough to even see the potential fun in the class. To make matters worse, the enthusiasm of the other participants left her feeling that they were handling their situations so much better than she. The contrast left her somewhat disappointed in herself because she was not coping better and also left her concerned that, because her predicament seemed so much worse than everyone else's, she truly did have cause for worry. How much those feelings contributed to what I found when I got home, I don't know. After greeting Laurie on the main level and being told Judy was asleep, I went upstairs, where I found Judy very awake and weepy and very sad.

Because I had thought and hoped we had turned the corner, I felt some frustration, even impatience as I held her. We talked for a long time, during which I got around to suggesting that maybe it was time to start diverting some of her focus away from her disease and the state of her physical body, and start doing other things. She wasn't alone, I reminded her. She had a good team of supporters around her to call upon when necessary. In the meantime, she needed to start occupying her mind and her time with some activities. In a short period of time we came up with drumming, different kinds of exercise, and even doing something with puppets. When we brought Laurie into the discussion, she enthusiastically lent her support and came up with a few more ideas, the result of which was that the ten days Laurie spent with Judy were pretty packed with activity.

Notable among the dinners, plays, visits with family and friends, babysitting Spencer, and dancing were some new and revisited activities. The day after the decision to do more, Judy tried doing a head stand, something she had previously mastered and done regularly in her yoga routine. Like riding a bike, it came back to her quickly, and she was standing on her head for a minute, minute and a half every morning. I'm not sure what benefits that is supposed to provide, but it certainly must give one a different perspective on life, maybe even turn conventional wisdom upside down. Also that day, Judy and Laurie went over to Annie's puppet theatre, where Judy got to act out a little of what was going on inside her. (That was also the time when she made public my alleged preference for the right breast, an accusation I feel I have sufficiently addressed earlier.) A couple of days after that, the three of us went to the health club when there were no classes going on. This allowed Judy the opportunity to try out some of the other activities, including slugging the big punching bag as long and as hard as she liked. Laurie also took her to a yarn store that day and then taught her how to crochet.

JUDY

The most amazing thing was how much "stuff" we did—we got out to plays, watched Spencer, had everyone over for dinner for our anniversary. I learned to crochet, tried a new set of exercises at the club, went out to eat several times, did puppet therapy with Annie, did a make-up class, drummed every morning, got back to doing head stands and decided to do them every day—already I can keep the pose for 90 seconds ... And so how did I still have time to get in funks and feel bad emotionally? Rhetorical question. The distractions don't always work because my mind goes back to what's happening in my body.

I needed to get my mind off that topic, and I found that mantras were helpful. I wrote out one mantra and put it on the refrigerator and every mirror in the house: "I choose to have an aura of abundance." Later I used "Breathing in health, breathing out the dying cancer" and "Energy Now." I thought of these mantras when I needed to relax and get through difficult moments. When focusing on an entire phrase became overwhelming, I just focused on counting. It kept me grounded and passed the time. I also pictured myself being held in someone's arms or being swayed in a hammock, and that often was the last thing I recalled before I fell asleep. How many strategies are there for soothing oneself? I seemed to need more and more of them.

Naps during treatment were very necessary. My body was worn out, and my emotions were raw. Nap time became a neutral zone; when I slept, I could believe that I didn't have cancer. Medical professionals encouraged me to nap: they said, "Cells regenerate best while a person is sleeping." I enjoyed continuing with naps well beyond my early recovery days. Fortunately, I have a flexible enough schedule to permit them. I recently found a quote of Winston Churchill's in which he promotes and defends naps: "You get two days in one, or at least one and a half." That's how I feel. With a nap, I can experience wake-up energy twice in twenty-four hours.

The only one of my previous activities that became even more important during treatment was the Dances of Universal Peace. Back in September 2001, shortly after the 9/11 attacks, I discovered the dances, a gathering of people who share a need and commitment to communal experiences that generate peaceful energy to send out into the world. A participant can take the dances on many different levels (in other words, it's an opportunity to move, an opportunity to socialize, an opportunity to nourish the spirit, an opportunity to sing); all are worthy, and all are gratifying. For me the dances were an opportunity to sing and dance—to recapture the joy I felt when I did those things in childhood. The dances were also an opportunity to develop a greater awareness of community and our roles in it—to connect with others who value coming together with people from diverse walks of life for the purpose of affirming peaceful practices in local and global interactions. Most of all, the dances brought me joy, calm, and optimism. There were few Wednesday nights, even during the worst of the treatments, when I did not get to the dance. No matter that I wasn't able to drive myself there, or that I wasn't able to stay for the whole event, or even that I danced at a slower pace. Fellow dancers were just the people I wanted to be surrounded by when I was in need; they are very caring. Perhaps yoga should have been as pleasurable, but yoga was more isolating, and I very much needed the community the dances provided.

DAN

It all seemed to be going well enough. Throughout Laurie's visit, once the activity emphasis had been decided upon, Judy had only one crying spell. Most of the time she was too busy, and then too tired, to dwell on her cancer. It was also approaching the end of the cycle; the effects of the previous chemo had diminished. That made it the best time to have so much going on, and Judy seemed to be taking advantage of it. However devastated she may have been by the treatment regimen, I saw that her instinct to seize every moment was still evident, an observation that was encouraging to me. Though her drive to pack the calendar usually made me nuts, and had caused a fair share of domestic squabbles over the years (me being the shy and retiring type), seeing her back in action was a definite relief. It was a hint that, yes, things might actually, eventually, get back to normal.

Judy's third AC treatment was on the day before Laurie was scheduled to return to Chicago. We all went to the infusion and then out to a Japanese restaurant for dinner. It was a quiet, reflective meal. We were glad to be in the moment, thankful for the positive turn of events of the past week, and grateful for Laurie's presence and support and the personal relief she provided. But we were also somewhat apprehensive about what might happen next. Would the next few days bring a repeat of the problems we had endured shortly after the previous treatment? It crossed my mind that maybe Laurie had come at the wrong time, that her presence would have been more valuable in the next ten days instead of the previous ten. One can always second-guess such a decision, especially after the fact. In one respect, it comes down to whether it is better to have a higher high or a more manageable low. But then the cycle was such that whatever came next totally obliterated the memory of what went before. One could only fall back on the dubious comfort of believing that things were just as they needed to be.

JUDY

There is a lapse in my journal of two weeks … two difficult weeks, as I write on February 14. *It was really hard to get any motivation to come to this writing place in the past two weeks. I'm not interested in writing here very often. I do it more or less out of a sense of duty, of knowing I will want to read this later.* There was a lot going on: side effects, visits and phone calls with family and friends, and a continuing agenda of trying to figure out how to handle the unpredictability of how I was feeling.

I also struggled with how to deal with all the encouragement I was receiving to rise above the physical misery I was experiencing. I couldn't simply dismiss these suggestions out of hand because not just them but the entire body of conventional wisdom said to "fight cancer—don't let it defeat you." Could so many people be wrong? I felt obligated to try it. I gave in to the peer pressure.

I decided to attend my Thursday-night book club. It was three weeks after my second treatment, so I hoped that I was past the worst of the side effects. Getting ready, in the quiet of my bedroom, I stayed positive, not allowing myself to dwell on the challenge the gathering might be. Being present with a group of friends eagerly talking to one another seemed appealing. I wanted to be there with them, to again be part of the life I had so enjoyed. Just thinking about it infused me with some energy. I went, determined to be part of the group and to show them how well I was doing.

Annie picked me up, and on walking in the door of Holly's house, I received a tremendously warm and supportive welcome. It felt great, and the euphoria should have carried me through the evening. But it didn't, and I couldn't pretend otherwise. Not long after my grand entrance, I retreated to a corner of the couch and wished I could become invisible. I wanted to ask Annie to take me home immediately, but I didn't want to ruin her evening or alarm my friends. I stuck it out, suffering in silence, detached from the group. The smell of the food nauseated me. I could not bring myself to eat it, yet I knew it was sumptuous. Then I felt assaulted by all the talking, overwhelmed by my friends' normal conversational voices. What they were saying should have interested me, but instead it oppressed me. I couldn't kid myself or others; it hurt too much to be there.

Or anywhere. I couldn't fight my way through this. I wasn't any good as a fighter. It took too much energy to fight, and all my energy was being used to endure, to wallow, and to worry. I needed a different way to deal with everything. The usual ways weren't working for me.

Per the previous pattern, the third treatment happened on Tuesday, and by Sunday I was wiped out. By Monday I was my weepiest. *I had expected to feel up to taking the car in for service and going to Qualife, but when I woke up, I felt lousy. So I cancelled the car service and called Chris, who graciously agreed to treat me.* (Chris had been a previous client in Qualife's Healing Buddies' program. When she had been in need, she received healing treatments, and now she was volunteering her services to give me Reiki treatments every week for six months. I treasured our time together, not just for the therapy, but for the conversation. I could bare my soul, and Chris was a gentle supporter.)

I enjoyed the treatment, but as she finished, I panicked and started sobbing hysterically. She sat with me, holding my hands, and talking about the difficult situation I was in (and that she had been in)—my tears were validated, as were my feelings. After Chris left, I left a message for Scotty. I calmed myself and stayed in bed. I didn't feel great but I got in control. Then Laurie called and I started all over with sobbing—"Nothing is working. I am feeling terrible. This is worse than last time." She gave lots of suggestions and support as best she could. As soon as I got off the phone with her, I reached Scotty and she said she could come right over. When I hung up from talking with Scotty, Cathlin called to see how I was and I started the tears all over again.

I might have expected to have "adjusted" to the effects of the treatment, this being the third one. But then again the effects change with each dose, usually becoming more intense. I sobbed to everyone I talked to that day, and I remember being fixated on how I no longer recognized myself (more internally than externally), that I felt a loss of my personality. I felt flat. The most comforting words that day came from a fellow survivor—"You *will* feel like yourself again when this is through." But there was little duration to the comfort, because it seemed I would never be through with this.

I told Dan and Scotty that I needed to have everyone around me and involved in my life. I must not be alone in this. I felt I needed to lean on other people's energy, since my own was so unreliable. I needed to be buoyed by their affection and attention. What I felt I could no longer provide for myself, I needed from others. I wanted to turn to the people I cared about for comfort, for hope, and for a connection to health, to confidence, and to capability.

When I made this known, everyone responded generously. Both of our sons offered their time and presence, and we called on all three sisters and many of our friends. I had never imagined being so needy, but I also never doubted that people could be counted on. It reminded me of that team-building activity—falling backward into someone's (hopefully) waiting arms to test your trust. My trust was high; with great confidence, I fell apart into those waiting arms.

DAN

The effects of the third treatment were initially marked by an extreme exhaustion that lasted almost a week. There were increased doses of anti-side effect medication, which might explain the fatigue. And the fatigue might explain the absence of any extremes in mood or anxiety, which returned on the sixth day.

When I got home from work that afternoon, Judy informed me that Scotty was on her way over to meet with us. Judy had arranged the meeting after crying herself through several conversations with friends that morning. When Scotty arrived, we sat in the living room. Judy informed us that she needed everyone to be more involved. Laurie's visit, regular sessions with Scotty, and my presence were great, but were not enough to overcome the dreaded and debilitating aloneness that descended on her when she was by herself. She could not continue that way. She needed people around her. She wanted Alex and Darren and their families more involved. She wanted to be with them often and regularly. She wanted her friends involved, always having someone with her. She wanted all her sisters to be with her. After she told us what she wanted, she instructed us to make it happen, and then she excused herself and went to bed.

I hadn't seen that coming. Suddenly she knew exactly what she wanted and was insistent that she get it. I was so taken aback that I didn't even have a chance to register disappointment—disappointment that the steps we had already taken were not enough. But it was easy to see that those steps had probably triggered her request. Her time with Laurie and Scotty had given her a taste of what she needed. Because companionship felt right, it only made sense for her to want to immerse herself in more of it.

Scotty and I talked for a while. We talked about the logistics of honoring her request, but we did not discuss the merits of it. In retrospect, I find that interesting. I would still have trouble debating whether there was a downside to surrounding her with people. Whether her request was a product of a trying moment that might change with the passage of a few hours or a few days also was not something to argue. She was very emphatic and clear about what she wanted, and the only question left to us was how soon and how completely we could make it happen. That we might be arranging a long-term solution to a short-term problem was beside the point. Getting it all done quickly was the only priority.

Scotty did ask me about getting the boys involved more. It was odd that we hadn't to that point. They weren't unaware of what was going on, and there had been no avoidance on their or our part since the diagnosis. The seriousness and the permanence of what Judy was going through were hard to judge, and as a result we probably tried too hard to make it easy for our sons, or as easy as possible. In fact, we were probably doing what our parents had done to us, and what we swore we would not ever do to our children, and that was to protect them, shield them from our problems. We were still role modeling, putting on an illusory front that all was well and nothing was so bad that we couldn't handle it. There was no need to burden them with our "aging" issues when they were working so hard to build their own lives with their own families. They certainly didn't need to take on our problems, especially when it was only a small tumor, caught so early that it would only prove to be a damn inconvenience.

It was time to change that thinking. It was time to bring them in and call on their strength and their youth and their optimism. It was time to stop keeping them children by protecting them from the difficulties in life, and time to start honoring the adults they had become by asking them to help us face those difficulties. "How would they respond?" Scotty wondered. I had no reservations. They would be eager, and valuable, probably relieved to finally be a more integral part of what we were going through. I also believed the same would be true of the friends we would call upon. And of Judy's sisters.

Then Scotty asked me how I felt about this new approach. I suppose she was getting at whether I might see it as a failure on my part, that I was not able to get Judy through this on my own. And I suppose I was experiencing some of that, though at the moment that wasn't where my mind was focused. My response was more to the nuts and bolts of the arrangements, not the psychological aspect of Judy's request. "Oh, well." I stumbled around looking for a way to express what I was feeling. "I guess what it boils down to is that it's not my style. Some of Judy's friends, the ones I'll call to help out, are my friends as well, but some of them are hers, and I don't know them very well. So while I don't necessarily like to call anyone and ask for help, it will be even harder to call people I don't know well and try to arrange some kind of schedule. But it's just a style and comfort thing and certainly not a big deal in light of what it means to Judy. I'll get over it, and I'll get it done." And then with a laugh I added, "And Judy will have to deal with the long-term damage to my psyche when she's better and I have completely fallen apart. Right now it's all about her. My turn comes later."

But there was one problem I did have with the plan, and I don't recall if I shared it with Scotty at that moment, or at another time, or ever. Most likely I kept it to myself, because I knew it was something I needed to repress if I were going to be of any help to Judy. It was something I had noticed during Laurie's stay. I tend to be pretty vehemently introverted. Spending a lot of time with others, any others, wears me down and wears me out. I need time alone to recharge myself. Throughout the cancer ordeal, I could muster up whatever endless energy it took to be a positive help to Judy, because I knew that I could recharge myself while she was napping, which she did a lot. When Laurie was there, most of my alone time disappeared. I worked and then spent time with Judy, and then when Judy rested, the house was still not mine. I wasn't free to read or watch television or play computer games or cook or write or do a crossword puzzle. Someone else was in the house, so my time was not truly my own. Part of it was the sense that I had a guest to entertain. But that was only part of it—my hosting instincts simply were not very strong. The main part was that the visit was an ordeal for Laurie, as well. When Judy was not present, Laurie needed someone to either process it all with or to divert her from it. That's only natural and understandable, and I was happy to accommodate. It wasn't that I was forcing myself to fulfill some obligation in visiting with her. I have always enjoyed her company, and even beyond that I was grateful for any willing ears whenever I had the urge to rehash it all. It was not until she went back to Chicago that I realized how exhausted I was. And with the new plan of more and more people being around, I would have to find ways to better accommodate my own needs. But that was not the immediate issue. I first needed to arrange for all those people to be around.

JUDY

A cancer journey for a fifty-five-year-old is different from a cancer journey for a younger person, and one big difference is the maturity of one's children. Both our sons are grown and raising their own families. They live nearby, and we are close with one another. Dan and I knew my illness was hard on them—they had never seen their mother sick before, just as they had never seen their mother less than positive about everything. We also knew they would play a vital part in my well-being, and when directly asked to participate, they were creative and committed in their efforts. Both of them came with love, with open caring, and with lots of questions that were helpful in getting me to think of how to make things better and to reflect on my experience. They both showed compassion, understanding—I felt so loved and so loving of them. Both of them and their partners were a blessing to me.

My three sisters also chose to share my cancer journey with me. We had given one another support during our mother's cancer just six years earlier. That experience had made us knowledgeable about cancer, and during that time, we had talked at length about life and death, about communications and emotions. We hold similar values, above all a commitment to supporting one another. Each sister made a trip out to Denver from Chicago to spend time with us.

Debbie has always stayed as far away from medical talk as possible; my cancer experience was no exception. She came between my third and fourth chemo treatments, the first to arrive after my latest call for company. She was also the sister most distressed at seeing me in this condition—not my physical condition but my mental and emotional condition. She expected me to be the take-charge kind of person I was when Mom was sick and that I am in most cases. She thought I could have been more in control somehow. Neither of us fully understood how much I wasn't myself at that time. That visit disappointed both of us; in fact, it shook us up a bit, because we had always been close. She believed she would be better able to flow with a cancer experience, that such an experience is a natural pattern. My journey demonstrated differently. *The way I'm coping is not the only way to cope, but it is my way.*

Cancer is not a natural pattern, at least not the treatment regimen, and when the flow of life changes, the rules change. Or maybe there are no longer any rules on how to behave and react. Debbie's visit had left her unsettled and unsure of how best to contribute to the "support Judy" effort. She did contact Dan to make sure he was getting all the support he needed as my primary caregiver. Then, several weeks after her visit here, she sent me a treat package, a collection of amusements and pretty things to enjoy and contemplate. It was lovely to receive, and a sweet way to connect.

Laurie came back for the fourth and final AC treatment, because I needed the comfort of having someone else around again. This time her visit was scheduled to coincide with the worst of the chemo after-effects, when her presence would be most valuable. How grateful I was that she gladly agreed to take on the worst of it.

Bonnie, my third sister and the youngest, was also the one I had the most consistent communication with over the years. So Bonnie was always up to date on the medical and nonmedical details I dished out. She had visited for an extended weekend back in November, right after one of the early procedures when my cancer was still only going to be a "damn inconvenience." But she was the sister with children still at home and a demanding family business, so when I sent out my desperate call for company, she could not come until the end of March.

Finding ways to involve all the friends who wanted to lend support was very pleasant. Until I felt comfortable driving again, I needed transportation to appointments. That always meant a nice visit with a friend and a good lunch after the appointment. Here I was thanking them for their service to me, and they ended up thanking me for including them in my experience. And I just didn't wait for people to offer. I asked for help when I needed it. One especially bad day I called Annie, a friend and puppet master, and told her I needed "puppet therapy." I felt it would be a relief to put a puppet or two on my hands and get rid of some of the mind chatter I was dealing with. Annie and my sister Laurie joined me in donning puppets and speaking in different voices; it was a magical event. Soon after, Annie gifted me with a gorgeous fish puppet of my very own—a glittering jewel on a "magic wand"—to help me keep swimming.

My journey had a recurrent theme. I was so impressed with the many ways friends and family supported me that I kept thinking of how I could better support others when they might be in need. Receiving help was not uncomfortable to me at all, and it also made me realize how much others enjoy giving support. I sensed that I would be more generous and responsive when I had an opportunity to give.

Scotty often spoke of energy being finite. If we "waste" energy on worries, then we won't have energy available to celebrate, to be in the moment. That was a new perspective for me. Something in my nature says that worrying will prevent the worst from happening, so I have allowed worries to overwhelm me at various times in my life. But there was so much to worry about (real and imagined) in the midst of the chemo treatments, I began to want to give up worrying; it simply became too draining. I enjoyed reclaiming my energy and living more in the moment, realizing that none of us is guaranteed a certain length of life and that I could do better by seeking joy in each day I had, rather than worrying about how many more I might see. I began feeling less aversion to the roller-coaster ride. Each time there was a change of direction, I had greater confidence that I could deal with it—not fight it, but deal with it. On February 20 I wrote, *So much has changed in the last few days. I've been feeling good!* There went that roller coaster again.

The final AC chemo treatment occurred on February 24. While I had feared this last, most intense treatment, it actually turned out not to be the worst one. Perhaps just the fact of being done with the AC regimen was a relief. Laurie's presence, I'm sure, also contributed to the diminished impact. Within a couple of weeks my appetite was back, my energy was picking up, my thoughts were more peaceful, and my interest in doing things was budding.

On March 7 I wrote, *Now Dan seems to be feeling his well empty. As I waited for him to come up from downstairs so I could say goodnight, he got to the top of the stair railing, leaned his head on the banister, and said in a tired, sad voice, "I can't do this anymore." In the next breath he perked up and said, "Of course I can, and I will." And we hugged and I cried (perhaps he did, too)—I could understand how he was feeling. This is terribly hard on him. All I could manage to say was, "We're doing the best we can." And he agreed.*

Just the fact that I once again could notice and then respond to someone else's need suggested that maybe I had truly turned a corner.

DAN

It was no surprise how positive and accommodating everyone was when we contacted them about helping out. I believe people have an inner need to be needed, and being asked out of the blue to help so touches and so honors that need that people will relocate heaven and earth repeatedly for the opportunity to pitch in. So Darren arranged to spend every Tuesday with Judy until I got home from work. Alex decided that Judy would benefit from a support group, so they arranged to start going to one at Qualife every Thursday night. Debbie would come out for a five-day visit. Laurie would return for another week, but this time she would be there to help during the worst of the chemo treatment. Bonnie would make it to Denver at the end of March. Mary and Gail arranged to help out several times, as did a few other friends who accompanied Judy to assorted doctor or Qualife visits and usually arranged a lunch along with the trips. It surprised us how much everyone appreciated the opportunity to help. It was not unusual for the friends helping out to thank Judy for sharing her experience with them. Their thanks suggest that something more than friendship was going on. Certainly they were expressing appreciations to Judy for meeting their need to be needed. Perhaps they were also appreciating the opportunity to witness unknown territory, a place where they may be taken on an unwelcome journey themselves some day.

Still, all the sunshine everyone brought into Judy's life during that time somehow managed to cast a shadow or two in my direction. Since the day of the diagnosis, I had experienced moments of reservation regarding decisions made, how things were going, what was being done and what wasn't. As I have recounted several times already, I had my own instincts about what was right and what was best, but mostly I opted to keep them to myself, especially if they were radically different from how Judy was inclined. I knew that it was better to follow Judy's instincts. On more than a few occasions that was not easy, yet I managed to stick with my original decision to remain silent. Why? Prescience and chivalry were certainly part of the reason, but more of it had to do with an inherent insecurity regarding my own instincts. They didn't come with the conviction that accompanies knowledge and evidence. So on the issues of what would work for Judy, my instincts were simply not as valid as hers.

Deciding to unconditionally support Judy's instincts and decisions regarding her treatment was difficult. I was glad I made that decision early in the journey, and reinforced it every time I revisited it thereafter, but with the plan to invite in as much help as we could, I found that I was facing that decision yet again. Not for myself and my own instincts, but with those we asked to help. When we involved as many people as we could, we opened ourselves up to more versions of what was best, what was right, and what should at least be tried. Of course, not everyone put forth their take on what Judy needed. Most everyone arrived with exactly what was needed: love, support, and companionship. But enough people came to me, not Judy, with a definitive opinion about what we should or should not be doing. I felt I was continually reengaged in my original dilemma, deciding from countless options what might be best for Judy. Except instead of a well-repressed internal struggle out of the limelight, I now was forced to debate the merits with those who had answered our call for help. That, at best, was very uncomfortable.

Fortunately, the new struggles were not major battles. Mostly they were skirmishes—other people feeling they had to convey their impressions on how well Judy was, or was not, coping. And being the husband, the primary caregiver, I was also the liaison to the rest of the world—the press secretary, the point person. Everyone's unspoken assumption was that all such messages were to be routed through me. In turn, they expected me to respond to the inquiries and comments by tactfully reaffirming and re-explaining our chosen policy of strict adherence to the Western medical establishment's recommended response to cancer. Since this included enduring the worst that chemotherapy had thrown at us, it was not an easy policy to put a positive spin on. It immediately became apparent that I was not the best person to be on point. I'm pretty defensive by nature, as well as argumentative, and though I truly appreciated everyone's help, as well as the motivation behind their suggestions, I could not just let whatever they said go unanswered.

I don't think I became noticeably testy with anyone offering a sincere opinion, but I felt myself feeling that way internally at times. Some people opposed or were wary of the conventional medical approach, suggesting that Judy might have been railroaded into a treatment, or that a lack of initiative had forced her to simply submit to the cut-poison-burn approach that Western medicine has deemed the one right way to treat cancer. Others, less undermining, offered countless remedies, healing therapies, and people to talk to for comfort and understanding. I found myself having to defend and justify the treatment path Judy had taken and the support resources she had chosen. Then I had to explain why Judy was unlikely to take up what the person offered. It was just too overwhelming to try to incorporate anything more into the treatment. As best I could, I had to make it clear to everyone that I probably would not be passing along their opinions and suggestions to Judy. More importantly, I had to stress that the only thing that would work for Judy was what she believed would work—which, for better or for worse, was what the established medical profession recommended. That was Judy's choice. That was something I had to accept and adjust to, and I expected everyone else to support her by doing the same.

And now, having gone through the experience of having to manage everyone's version of "what's best," and having recorded it here, I wonder how Judy and I will respond to others when roles are reversed. I trust we will respond with what we found most helpful to us—something along the lines of unconditional support and flexible presence. But in reality, we will probably believe that we have the right answer, or at least a better one, and we will make sure whoever we are helping will get the benefit of our wisdom. What could be more natural?

Judy was rarely alone during the four weeks after she announced her I-want-more-involvement directive to me, with Scotty as witness, until March 6, when Laurie's second visit ended. Something was always going on, and someone was always there. That night, as I walked up the stairs to kiss Judy good night, I let the exhaustion overtake me. Unable to ascend the last stair, I threw in the towel, but even as I tossed it I remembered why I shouldn't, and I reached out to snatch it back. Fortunately, Judy was there to intercept it and hand it back to me. We were, indeed, both doing the best we could, and doing it our own way.

And things were beginning to work. The call for and the arrival of the cavalry seemed to make the difference. Though it was not an instant turnaround, and though we had days of feeling completely exhausted and miserable, the major dramatic episodes were behind us. There were no more anxiety attacks. No more emergency phone calls to health care professionals, no more early-morning or late-night visits to the hospital. Things had settled down, and when something physical became too insistent to ignore, we dealt with it, first with a calm acceptance and then with a certainty that it would pass, that it was a necessary by-product of the healing process. The fourth AC treatment produced its share of bad effects and resulted in us cancelling some plans, but the effects seem to be less intense—or, more likely, Judy was better able to deal with them. We were finally to the point where we could face further treatments without dread, where we believed any discomfort was part of the process to ensure the cancer was being dealt with as effectively as it could be. This was the point I thought—and hoped—we had been at two months earlier, when we so optimistically looked forward to the first treatment as the harbinger of longer and brighter days ahead. I think we must have been looking at the wrong calendar when we made that calculation.

10

The Merry Month of May

JUDY

Between the two rounds of chemo treatments, I wrote some startlingly upbeat journal entries. March 11: *I guess you would say I'm feeling happy this week—isn't it great to be able to carve out some happiness in the middle of this experience?* March 17: *I'm happy and enjoying myself and some of the time I forget my condition ... I'm feeling kind of normal like.* Also March 11: *People tell me the lilt is back in my voice.*

It was nice while it lasted, but it didn't last. The second round of four chemo treatments (Taxol) was not as debilitating as the AC round had been, but it wasn't a piece of cake, either. I was fine until the sixth day after the first treatment, when I sunk into a funk and then stayed tired for a few days. My thinking processes became slower and confused, and I found myself not taking on much that required clear-headedness. I felt more irritable, less likeable, and my patience was very thin. Some days I felt myself to be a switch that was in the "off" position and other days "on."

In early April I wrote, *I feel another layer of sadness. I am overwhelmed in public places. Since most of the time I am by myself in my own surroundings, I find the out-side world can be too much. When I'm out, I feel an over-stimulation that rocks my equilibrium.* One evening we went to our favorite bookstore and after about five minutes I needed to find a chair in a quiet place to calm myself. I thought going out would provide a nice distraction, but it only brought different anxieties.

Staying home wasn't a guarantee to feeling better either. In late April, two of my uncles came over for a visit. *I did not feel like their niece—I felt like their sister. I am twenty and thirty years their junior, but I am less healthy, less happy, and less confident than they are. I just feel very much out of my own at the moment. I've been believing that I was feeling better and getting through this better, but I am pretty much in a funk. My thinking is getting fuzzier, my fatigue isn't lessening, and I feel more irritable and less likeable. My patience is very thin in waiting for these next six to seven weeks to be over so that I might get a sense of really feeling better. The last two big treatments are on April 30 and May 21.*

The worst effects came with the first two treatments; the third and fourth were easier. But my nose continued to be drippy—I couldn't keep enough tissues in the house. And as had been the case with the AC, my fingertips were ultrasensitive and tingling. Finally, Taxol caused my few remaining hairs to fall out. The fact that hair loss made the list of worst Taxol side effects speaks to the lighter intensity of the second round of chemo. When dealing with the AC round, I had too much going on inside my head to be concerned about what was falling off it.

Coinciding with the first Taxol treatment, I also began my fifty-two-week regimen of Herceptin, a monoclonal antibody. The Herceptin regimen was part of a national clinical trial for breast cancer patients whose HER2/neu gene made recurrence more likely; 50 percent of patients received the drug, 50 percent did not. (When we initially visited with Dr. Caskey and heard the treatment possibilities, we made the choice to participate in the study and then had to wait a short while to find out if, in fact, I would be part of the randomized 50 percent who actually got the drug. I imagine it would have felt like another punch in the stomach if we were not selected, but that's the nature of clinical trials. Fortunately, the trial proved so effective that by summer of 2005 the trial part concluded and from that point on all participants were given the drug.) Herceptin required me to have my heart monitored. The test required me to lie still for a half-hour while machinery hovered over my chest. I did a baseline in December 2003 and retakes in March and September 2004 and June 2005. The tests always came back with good results.

Herceptin did not have any side effects, and so the challenge was mostly the idea of going to Dr. Caskey's every week for a year. At first that was overwhelming—just as thinking about seven weeks of radiation had been overwhelming—but after a while it became a comfort. It was like checking in every week with friends: I felt very supported.

Despite the occasional episode of roller-coaster riding, we were clearly getting to the end of taking strong medicine. And I was brightening just as spring was. I certainly took strength in the seasonal energy and beauty. In fact, I worked with a springtime visualization that was most encouraging. With guidance from Scotty, I pictured myself a year from the current spring. It was the first long-term projection I was able to make, and it was a breakthrough. *I felt deeply moved to picture myself embracing the chemo as powerful stuff and letting it do its work, the white cells rebuilding, the red cells rebuilding, and the cancer dying out and being flushed out, being pruned away. Then the normal cells become strong and pink again, and I am cancer free ... I am much relieved to be able to picture myself healthy again—to see a good outcome to this horror story. To feel some sense of lightness and laughter.*

One of the funniest moments came when I was fitted for my prosthesis in mid-February. Mary offered to accompany me to the fitting; neither of us could imagine exactly what that would be like, but I knew having her along would make it more pleasant. I had been told to bring an extra bra. The procedure was explained to us when we got there, and it was a unique experience to watch the technician at work, wrapping me and my bra in something like papier-mâché. Since I had to stand on my feet for a while, the technician kept reminding me not to lock my knees, to stay relaxed. But as she removed the cast from my torso and I felt this weird sensation of being liberated, I nearly keeled over in a faint. Whether it was a physical or emotional reaction, Mary and the technician almost had a body on the floor in that fairly small work space. No long-term harm, but quite a chuckle in retrospect.

A more telling moment came on my birthday (April 1). It fell on a support group night, and when I announced to the group that it was my birthday, the facilitator said that I would have to answer the standard birthday question: "What have you learned this year that you did not know the year before?" I blurted out a loud profanity as my immediate response, then explained my outburst. "That's a most awful question! Knowing I have cancer this year is not a happy learning." After a moment's thought, I was able to add, "But yes, I have acquired new resources; I am receiving support from many sources, and I am learning that I can cope with some awful experiences." The combination of feeling better and being in the support group helped put a positive, brighter spin on everything.

Another bright side, literally, was my red wig. Even before my short, wavy, black-hair-streaked-with-gray fell out, I had purchased a wig that looked very similar to my regular style. But once the hair fell out, I actually preferred wearing scarves for public appearances and a small cotton cap for around the house. At the next-to-last chemo treatment, though, I made a bold change. Gazing at the wigs in Dr. Caskey's office, wigs that previous patients had donated for others' use, Dan and I were attracted by a red wig. I didn't need any encouragement to try it on. Even without a stylist's adjustment, it looked good. It was straight, with bangs, and almost to my shoulders. We took it! The first time folks I knew saw me in the wig, they were startled. At a meeting I went to monthly, someone came over to me, thinking I was a new attendee. The wig had a positive impact on how I felt. Others commented on how much they liked it, and I took that to heart. It was fun to be different, to surprise people (and myself), and to look better. It also gave me the latitude to be lighter and freer. And six months later when my own hair started growing back, it was actually difficult to give up wearing the wig. For people who only knew me with the red wig, my black stubble was startling. We even toyed with the idea of coloring my hair red when it grew in; the wig had really given me a lift.

In early May, Scotty and I spaced our visits further apart—to every other week. By mid-May, I started swimming on a regular basis. That required shopping around for a bathing suit to accommodate my new figure. One small, positive step always led to another one. Life was getting fun again.

DAN

From my perspective, the crisis was over. Though Judy had another round of chemo coming up, one whose side effects we had not yet experienced, as well as the year-long clinical trial and at least one more major treatment surprise, by the time Laurie left ten days after the final AC treatment, I had no doubt things were going to get back to normal. Whether the cancer ever came back was no longer the issue. Surviving the treatment had been our focus. Cancer may have been the culture's bogeyman, but dealing with its cure was ours. Once it became clear that Judy was going to survive the treatment, the rest of the ordeal took on a lighter mood.

It is only natural to find the hysterical, the outrageous, the touching, and the bizarre in any such experience and then turn them into a collection of anecdotes to recount on numerous appropriate occasions for the rest of our lives. There is something about a medical crisis that seems to heighten one's perception of the details of the moment. An example of that occurred a few years earlier when Judy and I got the hopeless giggles in an emergency room while we waited for the X-ray report after I dropped a weight on my foot and broke three toes in five places. Nothing funny about that, but at the same time, we went into hysterics. What set it off was trying to visualize how our sex life might have to change without the full use of my toes. After trying to put that picture into words, everything was funny.

That spring, we had finally reached the hysterical point in Judy's medical crisis. For the five months since the diagnosis, nothing had been very funny. We were overdue for a good laugh and, sensing that, the universe responded. The only really funny moment to that point had occurred when Mary accompanied Judy to get measured for her prosthetic left breast. Since I wasn't there, I can only imagine how things got rolling then, but I was present when Judy picked up the prosthesis, and that turned out to be a pretty outrageous experience. Perhaps it was just the whole idea of going out to buy the kind of device that one would only expect to find in some adult arcade. "Looks and feels like the real thing," the advertising would proclaim. "Even has a nipple painted on it to match the color of the original."

The woman who ran the business was understandably proud of the product she had manufactured for Judy. She explained how to care for it and then spent an inordinate amount of time demonstrating how to glue it in place, pointing out the circumstances under which the glue would hold up, and where to get more glue when the initial supply was used up. Judy nodded and took it all in while I sat there in disbelief. Did the woman really expect Judy to glue the prosthesis on to a part of her body that was still restricted—too fragile, too tender, too haunted? But we listened to the instructions as if we intended to follow them. Then the technician put the device in place, and Judy modeled it for us. It was lovely. Shapely and firm. It was also an adolescent boy's fantasy: it was huge, at least by comparison with the original equipment on the other side of her chest. (And it didn't sag, either.) I didn't know whether to drool, or laugh, or complain that some boob at the boob factory had messed up the order. The woman rechecked the dimensions and said they were exact to the measurements she had taken when Judy first visited. Of course, that had been several weeks earlier, and with the rigors of the chemo treatments, Judy had missed a lot of meals and lost a lot of weight. "Oh well," Judy rationalized. "I'll guess I'll just have to put all those pounds back on. Poor me." The woman did tell us that, though unlikely, there were instances in which the insurance company would pay for a second prosthesis to accommodate a permanent weight loss. Judy told her that would be unnecessary. She figured she would have her figure back in no time.

But Judy never did use the glue. We left the prosthesis parlor with the device correctly glued in place. Whatever benefits of having it glued on were overshadowed that night when the removal process took an hour and a half. Granted, getting things off one's chest can be a difficult experience, but in theory there should be a cleansing sensation to accompany the act. The only cleansing that night came when we tried to remove the reluctant adhesive residue off the artificial breast and off Judy's skin. There was no way Judy was going to do that again. The whole idea of the prosthesis was to give oneself a normal and familiar look when dressed. The portable breast does that just fine when it is slipped into the empty cup. The point of gluing it on never became clear to me. If it was also supposed to give the illusion of normalcy when undressed, then there are so many things wrong with that aesthetically, philosophically, and practically, I wouldn't know where to begin. Suffice it to say that even the most realistically manufactured prosthetic breast and the world's greatest glue could not alter the reality of Judy's mastectomy—nor should it.

It also became clear after Judy started regaining weight that her right breast would soon grow to approximate the size of the artificial one. There would be no need for us to approach the insurance company for a second device to better adorn her new figure. Up to that point the insurance company had been very accommodating and easy to deal with, but it would have been awkward to push that claim, and maybe even a bit embarrassing if they accommodated us. And they might have. There seemed to be an unwritten rule that breast cancer victims get the no-hassle treatment from insurance companies. I often thought back to the Race for the Cure and figured those kinds of numbers represent a pretty potent constituency that legislatures and insurance companies readily acquiesce to. Fair or not, I got the impression this was the reality. And though we did not have a great insurance plan, it covered virtually everything. We had no problems. In fact, the company's willingness to cover everything created a crisis of conscience that we had to address once we got into the second round of chemo.

During the first round of AC treatments, Judy would go back to the doctor the day after the chemo (which she got on Tuesdays) to get a shot to boost her white blood count. This shot had to be given the day after the infusion. When we went to the Taxol round, we switched to our chemo appointment to Fridays for reasons that involved scheduling and seeing Dr. Caskey before the treatment. But Dr. Caskey's office was closed on Saturdays. This meant the shot to boost the white blood count either had to be given at the Infusion Center at the hospital, or I had to give it to Judy at home, or Judy had to give it to herself. Given Judy's pattern of relying only on health care professionals to treat her, there was never any consideration she would give herself the shot. And though I was willing, I was ruled out for the same reason. So after the first of four Taxol treatments, we went to the hospital on Saturday afternoon and got the shot, a process that took all of five minutes, most of which involved checking in and waiting. The shot took a matter of seconds. After the second treatment three Fridays later, we followed the same routine.

A few days thereafter, we received the explanation of benefits for the first shot. We were informed we were obligated to pay one thousand five hundred dollars. According to the explanation of benefits, that single, ten-second shot cost fourteen thousand dollars. With the hospital-to-insurance-company discount, the cost was reduced to a mere eight thousand dollars. Our share of that amount was three-quarters of our total out-of-pocket expenses for the year. Given the circumstances, there was never any question we would have to pay the full out-of-pocket for 2004 eventually. We just didn't expect to have to pay most of it at once and so early in the year. That was a bit unnerving. Naturally, we contacted the hospital and the insurance company and Dr. Caskey's office, absolutely certain that a gross mistake had been made. "No mistake" was the verdict from everyone, including the insurance company, which would be picking up the full tab on the remaining shots. It was outrageous. During the AC treatments, the cost of the shot had been covered by the basic office co-pay. The only explanation we were given was that hospitals overcharge when they can get away with it to maintain solvency. No one ever got around to saying that the medicine in that shot was really worth eight or fourteen thousand dollars. Its market price was determined by other means.

My outrage was not calmed, so rather than participate in a process that skyrocketed medical costs beyond reason, and even though it wouldn't have cost us any more out of pocket to go back to the Infusion Center, we decided that I would give Judy the shot after her last two treatments. The nurses had me practice with a syringe and a rubber ball while Judy was on the IV for her third Taxol infusion. I kept jabbing that ball, wondering if it really was similar to Judy's hip, where I would be jabbing the needle the next day. The nurses gave us the syringe, already filled, with instructions to keep it refrigerated until just before we used it. Looking at it, it didn't look to be worth eight thousand dollars, and definitely not fourteen thousand dollars. It was just a hypodermic with a little bit of something that was supposed to be good for Judy. I suppose I should have been nervous about dropping it or forgetting it was in the refrigerator when I put the pickle jar back. But I remained surprisingly calm, and when I got home from work that Saturday afternoon, I just did it. It was only a little nerve-wracking. My fears of not being able to penetrate the skin or breaking the needle off or the countless other things that could have gone wrong didn't materialize. I just gave her the shot and cheated the hospital out of eight thousand dollars. Judy was even kind, or tactful, enough to say it was the best shot she ever had. Three weeks later, we did the same thing. I was an old pro by then but refrained from discussing technique with the nurses at Dr. Caskey's office. I didn't want to give them the impression that I thought their job was easy.

It was at Dr. Caskey's office for one of the Taxol treatments that we discovered *the* wig. Judy, with her hairdresser's help, had gone out and had a wig made, one that closely resembled her natural hair and style. And it was fine in its own way. Judy always kept her hair too short and too curly for my taste, but that was a long-running disagreement that I was never going to win. My preference for the long, straight head of hair I had married was lost to convenience and practicality long ago. But in Dr. Caskey's office, many former patients had donated their wigs once their own hair had grown back, so there were always two or three for the current round of patients to choose from and take home if they liked. That day there was no one else receiving treatment, so it was just the two of us and the two nurses. I had dozed off earlier, as had Judy, but now we were both fully awake and I guess less than intrigued by whatever reading material we had brought with us to while away the three hours.

Looking around for something to amuse us, we noticed several wigs around the room, more than usual. There was no long, straight black one, so I asked Judy if she had ever wanted to be a blonde. My fantasies have never involved blondes, and I guess the same was true for Judy, because there was a decided rise in apathy when she emerged from the restroom as a blonde. But she had been sparked to try on new personas, and she grabbed a second wig, something in a nondescript, mousey brown and an unmemorable style. Not surprisingly, the impact was nondescript and unmemorable. Up on a shelf was a red wig. Not orangey-red or real red, but something in the auburn or chestnut family. The hair was straight, but not long, styled into something like an old pageboy, not unlike one of the ways Judy had worn her hair when we were young and falling in love with each other. The new color and the old style did it for me, and it worked for her, as well. When Judy walked out of the office that afternoon, wearing the wig, the young woman who worked the reception/appointment desk shrieked in delight and called her a hottie. I was not familiar with the term, no doubt an indication of my age and lack of television viewing, but I had to presume from the woman's expression and usual sincerity that "hottie" was, like, totally complimentary, even when applied to a single-breasted gal in her midfifties. I have always thought of Judy in that way, though I never used that exact term, and I did not start using it then. But being a hottie was a nice change of pace. So was being a redhead. She never again wore the wig she had bought, always opting for the more fun red one. And when her own hair grew back, she chose not to return the red wig to the doctor's office for someone else to use. It had earned a special place in her life, in our life—a reminder of when life started being fun again.

We had some fun with Laurie, too, when she was helping out for Judy's last AC treatment. We were having Darren and Alex and their families over for dinner, both to see them and in honor of Laurie's presence, as if she were a regular out-of-town guest just paying us a visit. It was, in fact, Laurie's fiftieth birthday that day, though none of us had mentioned it yet. We intended that night's dinner to be a celebration, and if the subject of birthday did not come up in the course of the day, then it would be a surprise party, as well. It helped us set the stage for a surprise when Laurie asked how she could help us prepare for the gathering. We suggested she bake a cake for dessert. She worked on that while Judy and I went out shopping. When dinner was finished that night and Laurie brought the cake to the table, we stuck a candle in it, lit it, and sang happy birthday. Then we gave her the gift we had bought for her that afternoon while she was in the kitchen baking her own birthday cake.

A few weeks later, during Bonnie's visit, we filled the house again to celebrate Spencer's first birthday. And about a week after that we gathered everyone once more, this time for Judy's birthday. These were not new, seize-the-moment kind of events for us. It was simply getting back to what we had always done. But Judy probably celebrated with a renewed enthusiasm. She was the one who, having been threatened with losing such times, gained a renewed appreciation for the value of each and every moment. For me, getting back to normal was more relief. I had never considered that these special times were limited, only that they were on hold for a while. I was more relieved that we were able to enjoy them again.

In addition to the family gathering, Mary took Judy out to lunch for her birthday, and they spent part of the afternoon together. Afterward, based on that time together, Mary e-mailed Judy asking if she had done something wrong, because Judy had seemed so distant while they were together. Judy told me about it, concerned that she might have inadvertently given a wrong impression. Judy tried to contact her, but they missed connecting several times. In one of those telephone-tag attempts, I found myself on the phone with Mary. We talked about the situation for a while, and I assured her that I still got the same distance from Judy on a fairly regular basis. I would cook a favorite meal only to have it pushed around on the plate. Plans for a walk would be cancelled in favor of a nap or would be taken, but without any conversation. She was still in the midst of the Taxol treatments, and often the accumulation of things took her over and simply zoned her out. As ready as we all were for the old Judy to be back, and even though she showed more and more flashes of being back, she simply was not there yet. We were maybe a little impatient and a little anxious to have this cancer thing in the past, but it wasn't going to hurry up for us.

JUDY

On May 21, I had my last chemo treatment. What a celebration! The oncology team feted us with balloons and a certificate and a photo to mark the occasion. And the doctor mentioned how pleased she was to see how I had "blossomed" since the low times of early treatment days. Dan and I celebrated with a brief mountain getaway, the highlight of which was a long hike. Dan was thrilled "to have me back." And I was beginning to think of other things besides cancer treatments. I had a sense of rediscovering myself and of rebuilding my world.

Yet, as good as I was beginning to feel, I wanted to protect my reflection time, my slower pace, and my choice of doing only things I really wanted to do and being with people I wanted to be with. *I have no interest in putting too much on the calendar—there is too much to savor … I have enjoyed the more reflective pace that cancer gave me.* Dr. Schewe would ask me almost a year later, "What helped make you a survivor?" And what came to me as a response was that I had needed to make my world smaller during treatment and then slowly grow it bigger again. I kept it manageable; I didn't play Superwoman.

Then, as if it were scripted and knew just when to make its reappearance, my work picked up. As my energies improved and I began to think more to the future, work came my way, even without my actively seeking it. The time was right. Work had taken a backseat, or no seat at all, for almost six months. Being self-employed gave me the freedom to make my own schedule, but it also affected our income. We made do. I didn't want to work when I felt poorly; I didn't want to pull myself together to do something for someone else, especially when I lacked confidence in my abilities. I did, however, enjoy one work-related activity during the worst of the treatments. I purged files. I got rid of old baggage in the work arena. Perhaps it was an early sign of my cancer, but I had become cranky with several clients during the few months prior to my diagnosis. With a respite from concentrating on work, I saw that wrapping up and walking away from those projects was what I needed to do.

About the same time, and this was definitely not scripted, I began to put on weight. *I am putting on the weight I lost. For a while I just ate whatever I wanted, and now I think I need to be less indulgent. It would be nice to keep off ten pounds or so. Wonder how quickly my taste buds will feel "normal" again? Food is indeed a comfort now.*

My biggest difficulty after chemo was in dealing with the fact that I looked so different than I used to. When I saw photos of myself in pre-cancer days, I was amazed at how good I looked—young, vibrant, happy. *I feel like I look older now and more serious and definitely not as attractive … A bit startling how peaked I look. My eyes are vacant, my lips not as full, my cheeks sunken.*

As I started to recover, I also felt a powerful, positive sensation. My gosh, I survived that awful experience! My worst fears had not been realized, and the experience didn't last forever. (I recognize that I was fortunate to have a treatable cancer.) It was not quite a feeling of being "Superperson," but it was quite amazing that normalcy returned. And that I was able to recognize a lot of learning experiences (gifts, if you prefer), which were wonderful ramifications of going through such a time. Gratitude tops the list, of course. But there was much more. I felt as if I gained more peace and patience, stronger intuition, and greater acceptance and appreciation. I was able to redefine my quality of life. I had been able to deal with ambiguity. I was resilient. The crisis of the moment had stimulated changes, but not only temporary ones. It is amazing and inspiring to learn what we can cope with, even if we fall apart during the journey.

While I was learning, I also was teaching others, and that concept was pretty powerful. My preference for telling it like it is has helped others learn about the mysteries of disease and how they might deal with it. Scotty often told me during our sessions that I taught her. At the time I didn't ask how or what, but just hearing her comment was affirming. When later I asked her for details, she said she had learned that our authentic self is sometimes the greatest gift to others. That was certainly how I saw it! She also said that in sharing my journey she had been reminded of how important it is to encourage the expression of emotions. "Emotions are the lubricant for our journeys," she observed.

In the beginning, when we were in a crash course with medical professionals, I read a lot of information about other people's cancer journeys and other professionals' advice for people on cancer journeys. Most would say that cancer is life-changing in a positive way. Simply put, "You have to give up something in order to receive." Before having actually gone through such an experience, those words are not very helpful; they sound terribly trite and self-servingly noble. And yet, once we have completed a difficult journey, we can't help but want to value it, celebrate it, and learn from it. It's a matter of attitude as to whether or not we recognize the gifts that we get from hardship. For me, there was no question of whether or not I would recognize the gifts. I was back to my "old" self, and my old self was an appreciator, a celebrator, a valuer. How could I not acknowledge that what I had just been through had had positive consequences, in addition to a return to physical health?

DAN

By the time the last Taxol treatment came in mid-May, Judy's bad days and most of the zoning-out episodes were gone. The only lingering effect seemed to be her need to rest regularly, including a serious afternoon nap. That, and a more deliberate pacing, distinguished the new Judy who celebrated the end of chemo.

We used the occasion to take an extended weekend in the mountains, spending three nights at a lodge in Grand Lake about a week before the tourist season got into full swing. Except for a modest art fair going on that weekend, we pretty much had the town to ourselves. Our first morning there we hiked into Rocky Mountain National Park. It was a manageable route, meaning not much elevation change, which probably contributed to our going on long past the time limit we had set for ourselves when we started. Judy was energized by the scenery and by being outdoors and taking part in a familiar activity again. We hiked to a waterfall, where we rested for a bit, deciding the increasing steepness of the trail made it a good place to turn around. It turned out to be a seven-mile hike, the distance only important in the sense of accomplishment it afforded us. Judy was more like her old self, and it wasn't just optimism and wishful thinking making that claim. There were seven miles of evidence behind it.

Of course, she slept away most of that afternoon, recuperating from the hike. I used the time to do what I usually like to do on vacations: nothing. I got a cup of coffee and a place to sit and watch that particular part of the world go by. And when I got tired of that, I set up the laptop and got to work on a novel, a ghost story I had started a couple of years earlier and was getting back to for another serious effort. When Judy got up, we went into town for some dinner and then hung around the lodge drinking hot chocolate and watching night descend on the lake.

We followed that pattern the next day as well: modest activity in the morning, followed by lunch and Judy's nap, during which I vegged out for a while and then returned to writing. It was a dream time for me, but Judy also got around to acknowledging what a great way it was to spend a vacation. She now understood why I always preferred it to her way, which was to fill up and take advantage of every moment in doing or seeing something special. It was nice to hear her appreciate what I had always known and lobbied for, usually unsuccessfully. There was warmth in that validation. But I also knew as she said it that she would soon be back to her customary ways. Not on that particular trip, but the progress back to who she had always been was rapid and undeniable. The cancer patient who had occupied her for several months was being exorcised.

11

Summer of R&R: Radiation and Reflection

JUDY

On my first checkup at Dr. Caskey's after the last Taxol treatment, we heard that we might not be as done as we thought we were. Yes, I would be coming in for an infusion of Herceptin every week for nine more months, but now we were looking at the likelihood of radiation. I was irritated to hear that. I thought radiation was unnecessary, given that I had had a mastectomy. But Dr. Schewe explained that since chemo traveled via the blood vessels, and my blood vessels had been compromised by the mastectomy, doing radiation would be added insurance against a recurrence. Radiation is site specific and will get any remaining cancer cells in the surgical area. I understood the logic but was disappointed not to be finished. I no longer viewed radiation as the equivalent of a life sentence; I was now less intimidated and felt able to manage a mere seven weeks of five-days-a-week visits. It is all what you have to compare it with, and after chemo, almost anything else sounds good.

Radiation actually had perks. There were donuts and jigsaw puzzles in the waiting area, and only five minutes of actual treatment, during which I could stare at an aesthetically-pleasing photo of aspen trees on the ceiling. And on top of all that, there was the comfort of being on a regimen and the satisfaction of knowing I was doing the most and best I could to get healthy again. I even overcame my fear of touching my scars and my unfeeling skin by having to put cream on that area four times a day for nearly nine weeks. I only got a mild burn from the treatments, and I enjoyed my indulgence in afternoon naps. *How quickly seven weeks went by,* I wrote on August 28.

DAN

Just as we were heading to the end of the chemo, Dr. Caskey threw us a new wrinkle. She had presented Judy's case to some panel of cancer experts, which I believe had the totally uninspired, and actually tasteless, name of The Tumor Board. The TB met to discuss interesting and/or unusual and/or instructive cancer cases and make recommendations to the presenting doctor—that is, when they weren't, I imagine, oohing and aahing over the specifics of the case. Why Judy's case was selected, I am not sure. Her case was certainly highly unusual, interesting, and instructive to us, but I never thought of it as having a more universal appeal (until we were encouraged to write this book). Obviously Dr. Caskey felt Judy's cancer had the elements that suited it for presentation, and the ensuing discussion resulted in the recommendation that once the chemo was done, Judy should go through a complete round of radiation treatment.

If, just a couple of months earlier, radiation had been thrown into the game plan, it would have been another crisis. We would have seen it as a potentially back-breaking straw, adding an eternity to what was already an interminable process. It might have also fed Judy's unhealthy perception that something was going wrong with the treatments; why else would they be adding a new treatment? But at the end of the second round of chemo, and settled into the weekly Herceptin infusion, we went to see Dr. Schewe, the radiation oncologist, curious and still open-minded, yet also ready to say enough is enough. After all, they had cut the tumor out and then poisoned Judy for five months just in case any shred of it remained. Now they wanted to burn the remaining landscape, on the off chance the cancer had any thought of picking itself up on its feet and having another go-round. It seemed like overkill, but we were in a state of mind that if Dr. Schewe had a good rationale, we would go along.

And, of course, he did. These doctors are good. The chemo, the rationale went, was delivered via the bloodstream and, therefore, would only be effective to areas where blood circulated. When the mastectomy was done, the circulation in that area was compromised, making it possible that not all areas where the left breast had been had received the full potency of the chemo. Since that is where the cancer was, it was important to be sure that everything there was treated. Hence, radiation was recommended to make sure the coverage was complete.

That was a good argument. We agreed to the recommendation. Looking back, I am not sure the rationale was all that tight. What bothered me was that, if there was no circulation to the area where remaining cancer cells might be hiding, wouldn't the lack of circulation, with its accompanying nutrients, doom those cells anyway? If they were there and getting circulation and nutrients, they would also be getting the chemical poison, wouldn't they? If they weren't getting the circulation, they would die anyway. Unless, of course, cancer cells somehow exist without the basic necessities of life other cells need. I'm no expert, and even if I had raised the question back then, almost any answer would have satisfied me. Even now I am not motivated to find out. In the big picture, it was not about being right. At that point, it was about a little bit of extra insurance. Five treatments a week for seven weeks was a low enough premium to pay for the added sense of knowing that we had done everything possible to make sure Judy was cancer free.

Radiation brought its own set of side effects, though none were as severe as what came with the chemo. The skin could burn, like a bad sunburn. The treatment could cause fatigue. Judy did not experience either to any great extent. Toward the end of the seven weeks, her skin was showing some redness. As for feeling fatigued, well, the routine of having to get herself to the radiation oncologist every Monday through Friday was draining in and of itself. But Judy was emerging from a six-month altered state, so having the reason to get up and go out returned her into a familiar mode of activity. She walked a mile to catch the bus to the radiologist and then had a mile walk on the return trip. It was actually a nice way of getting back into her life.

JUDY

I had thousands of moments of reflection during my cancer journey, and I relished them. In fact, sometimes I intentionally chose activities that allowed me time for reflection. Like my trips to radiation. My pleasant pattern was to walk a mile to catch a bus, take a fifteen-minute bus ride, have my five-minute treatment, stop for a cup of coffee, catch the return bus, and finish with another mile walk. Fortunately, I went through radiation during the summer months, so weather was not an issue. Riding the bus had benefits. I could let my mind wander, and I could observe other people and scenery. And as I got to be a "regular," the bus driver became friendly. (At the end of my treatment weeks, I felt I needed to alert the driver not to look for me any more. I didn't want him to worry.)

Reflection time quiets the chatter in your head, allows you to escape from unpleasant thoughts, and grounds you in the moment. The mind seems to become more fertile, more intuitive, and contentment is easier to access. Over the course of my treatment and recovery, I grew increasingly comfortable and appreciative of my own powers of reflection. (As I write these words, I have just read *The Alchemist* by Paulo Coelho, who wrote, "Reflection time allows you to hear your heart." I like that description. My heart has a lot to say to me; I imagine everyone's does.)

But while reflections are enough in and of themselves, they are even better when they are shared. By sharing them, I got the opportunity to clarify them, to let them deepen and take root. I had my journal in which to record them, and I had Dan to listen to them in whatever unformed state they might be. I also had family and friends to share them with, and along the way I found Scotty. Also along the way I found the support group at Qualife, where I not only got to share my reflections but received the benefit of many others caught up in similar circumstances.

We discovered Qualife as a family: each of us participating in some Qualife activity. My initial interview there was one of the most affirming encounters of my cancer journey. After hearing all about me, the counselor said, "It sounds like you have much in your life that contributes to your well-being." Qualife had many program offerings: art workshops, drumming workshops, weekend retreats, nutrition workshops, support groups, individual counseling, and body therapies.

At the beginning of my cancer experience, support groups were not an option I wanted to consider or even talk about. That was odd, because I have always been a very sociable person, someone who believed in the strength of sharing, and someone who was a joiner. But I was adamant that I didn't want to attend a group effort in which I would have to hear other people's horror stories. And the first such groups I heard about didn't appeal because they were held at the hospital—I had had enough of the hospital, even if the rooms were warmly decorated.

But amid the flood of tears that characterized the first two months of chemo, our son Alex convinced me to try a support group. He offered to find a good one and be my transport and companion. I put the logistics in his hands. Qualife had several support groups, and since I was already enjoying the Healing Buddies program, he tried there. The breast cancer group had just started a new eight-week session and preferred not to admit any latecomers. I understood. The next one was starting in another eight weeks, but it didn't make sense for me to wait for that opportunity. The other options were either a women's cancer group or a coed cancer group. Because I wanted to share the experience with Alex, we chose the coed cancer group. It was the right group for us, and my mindset did a 180-degree turn regarding support groups. At the first session we attended, I heard cancer patients and their families and friends laughing. Imagine that! I heard people sharing stories similar to mine, but they were further along in treatment or recovery, and I found their stories inspirational. I was at the lowest point in my own experience the night I joined the group, but within several weeks I had refilled my well, and I began to contribute more than my tears. Alex accompanied me as often as he could; Dan came when Alex couldn't.

I commented to another cancer patient about my feelings for support groups, after I had been in the Qualife support group for a while. "We all rationally know we are not alone in our experiences," I said, "but we can trick our minds into thinking we are alone unless we actually meet and hear (and learn) from folks who are also on this unwelcome journey."

The experience for Alex (and also for Dan) was rich. Here Alex was meeting and being a peer with older people who were dealing with something totally out of his scope of experience. The knowledge he gained about medicine, about coping, about not coping, about what's important, etc. was a treasure trove. And he contributed as much as he received. Before we went, he thought he was merely going to accompany me, but from the first night it was clear that each of us, individually, was getting something special and something needed out of the group experience.

In hindsight, I am grateful that I was part of this group that dealt with such a variety of cancers and that brought together diverse people. I believe it was through our work with Qualife that we were able to ease ourselves into radiation treatments, even though that addition to the treatment plan was dropped on us unexpectedly. With the example of how so many others handled a variety of treatments, we were much more confident and prepared to adjust to the change. Yes, I could have received benefits from an all-women's group or a breast-cancer-only group, but the bigger picture in the general coed group helped me to integrate myself with others in the world.

I remember one poignant evening at support group when the husband of another patient asked Dan how he dealt with his new role as caregiver. He relayed something he had told me earlier and told anyone who asked him how he was dealing with it: "When we married, we knew, whether we acknowledged it or not, that one day one of us would need the other's caregiving." When I was diagnosed, he stepped into that role comfortably and eagerly. To do otherwise was not even a thought.

I must note here that Qualife closed its doors in December 2004, ten months after we fell in love with it. That was very sad for us and many others; we felt that a resource like Qualife added immensely to our well-being. Here's what I wrote about Qualife in preparation for a newspaper interview at its closure.

The support groups have been amazing, wonderfully inspirational. Every time we leave a session we are awe-struck by the depth of conversations we just had, by the witnessing of people's abilities and needs, by the coming together of a community of strangers into a community of caregivers. Our own feelings of optimism are fed, as is our confidence and gratitude. We are treated with gentleness, respect, understanding, and humor; these sessions helped me to laugh again. Staff are excellent role models for us participants—we develop our own skills of compassion and listening and self-awareness … Cancer is a complex journey; it affects all aspects of our lives, not just our body. It's a horrible roller coaster, a long-term challenge with many phases. We need resources for the other parts of our lives—especially our emotional and social needs. We need a TEAM: a community of diverse people. We need to be able to bring our whole selves someplace. We need a PLACE other than medical offices. Our caregivers, families, and friends need resources and support—it's not just about us patients. That's what Qualife is, a community.

Another topic of reflection for me was what I perceived to be my increased patience or empathy. *I like the peace and patience that I seem to carry now. I know it is a result of this year's cancer journey, and I'm grateful for those gifts. I like my acceptance and appreciation of a greater variety of people. I like and trust my intuition; it feels stronger.* The experiences at Qualife no doubt contributed to this growth.

There are so many breast cancer resources that it can be overwhelming to decide which ones to tap into. As Dan noted, the incredible success of Race for the Cure stimulated the creation of a plethora of assistance for patients and their families and friends. Day of Caring (Colorado) puts out a directory of breast cancer resources every year—a listing of more than fifty pages. There are local organizations, national organizations, and Web site organizations; there are products, information, help lines, support groups, exercise groups, counseling, makeup sessions, and much more. I appreciated having such choices and opportunities, but I didn't drive myself crazy trying to benefit from all of them. When I felt a new need, I'd look for a new resource.

The summer of radiation and reflection came and went. My eyebrows and eyelashes returned with great speed. So did my mustache—the good with the not so good. Time to get out the bleach again! My hair had grown back just enough to start covering the ugly spots on my scalp, and by mid-September I retired the red wig. I didn't pursue coloring my returning hair red, but I felt an insistent need to put more color into my life. That's when I turned my attention to our bedroom walls. They were begging to be enhanced. Since it was a very light room with plenty of sunshine, I dared to paint the walls a deep purple. And the results were very pleasing. Plus, I got to enjoy the sheer fact of doing some physical labor.

DAN

A combination of things made the additional summer of treatment easy to accept and easy to do. Mostly it was the absence of chemo. Not being physically sand-bagged every three weeks would make most anything feel doable. In fact, Judy probably felt a pent-up need to get out and do something with that resurrected sense of capability. Going to radiation happened to come along just when Judy needed to get back in a routine. But her renewed energy alone did not necessarily make traipsing off every day for more cancer treatments an acceptable activity. Judy had to also be emotionally ready to endure the unplanned extension of her engagement with cancer. She was in that ready state due to her ongoing involvement with Scotty and to her participation in the Qualife support group.

I cannot speak to the specifics of how working with Scotty helped Judy get past the debilitating fears that had brought her so low. Certainly Scotty was a sounding board and a catalyst for the steps that turned the situation around. As the first cavalry scout to come over the hill, she taught us that reinforcements were probably a good thing, and the more the better. Being open to more is what led us to Qualife.

Judy and Alex began going to the support group at Qualife in February. Judy was at her lowest point when she started, and she reportedly cried her way through her initial meeting. But when she got home she had much to tell me about: the people, their situations, the facilitator, and, of course, how much she had cried. She also told me Alex had contributed significantly to the group, and that he seemed to get a lot out of his participation. It was just a good experience in so many ways. I couldn't disagree, though from my perspective I must admit I most appreciated having the night off. Still, I became a little curious about the group.

My curiosity was satisfied the first time Alex could not go, and I went as his substitute. It was not a requirement of the group that someone be there with Judy—it was more that Judy preferred to have someone with her. When the reality of going was presented to me, my curiosity ran directly into my negative instincts regarding such groups. But since it was still all about Judy at the time, I kept my poor attitude to myself. Unfortunately, and as if by design, the first part of the session reinforced my negativity about the value of such gatherings. I am not a group person anyway, as I'm sure I have already mentioned. On top of that, I am also not one who appreciates mental visualization, guided or otherwise, therefore I also don't get much out of it. So when the group started out with self-introductions, I was immediately overcome with all the usual hang-ups I have about speaking in front of a group, an affliction that always inhibits my ability to listen to what anyone else is saying. I don't exactly remember what I said to introduce myself, but I think it was the first time in Judy's whole cancer experience I heard myself referred to as a caregiver.

Once that part of the group ordeal was over, the facilitator made it worse for me by leading the group in a guided visualization, meant to relax us and make us feel good. We were to escape in our minds to an extra-special spot. I tried, but mostly I was very much stuck in my chair at Qualife. I frantically tried to imagine myself by a river in the woods, or on top of a mountain, or in a coffee shop down the street. I flitted between the three at such a pace that I completely missed the relaxing aspect of the exercise.

The painful obligatories out the way, the discussion turned to a new member of the group. She was asked to tell her story, and as she did I was reminded of the other reason I avoid this kind of support group. If you need support, why look for it in a place where everyone is looking for the same thing, where each tale of woe out-woes the one just told? Does the support come from the fact that hearing someone else's worse predicament makes you feel better? Is that support? Or comfort? That's taking the theory of relativity a bit too far for my taste. If I can only feel better by comparison, because someone in the same room as me is doing worse, then the relief can only be temporary; most of my life will be spent away from the support group, where my tale is much more woeful than those around me.

As I listened to the newcomer relate her circumstances, I found myself thinking there was nothing of comfort to say to this person. She was un-partnered in life, economically unsuccessful, and her only son, a young man in his early twenties, was dying of some kind of cancer. The details were more horrific and went on and on, but that was the gist of her tale. The group was pretty much silenced as the woman finished and waited for a response, maybe even dared anyone to try to offer some comfort. She had nailed it, and had we been on the show *Queen for a Day*, she would have walked away with the new refrigerator. The facilitator of the group broke the silence by thanking her for sharing her story. Then she asked the woman what she saw as positive in the experience. The question naturally surprised the woman. Of course there was nothing positive in it, but the question obviously unsettled her. Rather than reiterate the negatives, which she had to believe the facilitator had somehow missed, the woman struggled for a response.

Finally, she jokingly said something about how she and her son were spending a lot of time together, but her sarcasm was evident. The facilitator's question, however, roused the rest of the group, and all of a sudden, everyone had something to say, picking up details of the woman's tale and showing how, from a slightly altered perspective, she could view some things as positive.

By the end of the session, I understood why Judy and Alex were so upbeat and so loyal to this group. It brought out something in everyone—probably that need to be needed—and in so doing, everyone was more articulate, more insightful, more understanding, more human, and more healthy than when they had walked into the room, including me—and I'm not even sure I contributed anything to the discussion. Yet I knew when I left that night, I wouldn't mind if Alex had to miss another night so I could return. But while it made a believer out of *me*, the woman never returned to the group, which could simply mean that she got everything she needed in that one session and could handle her circumstances better because of the experience.

I understood that I could have gone to the group anytime I wished. I didn't need Alex's absence to open up a spot for me. But meeting for dinner and then going to Qualife every Thursday night had blossomed into something more between Alex and Judy. It was special time together for them, just as Judy's Tuesday mornings with Darren had been during the tough, early chemo treatments. My presence would naturally change the dynamics, and while that would not necessarily be a bad thing, it would be different. For Judy, it was a rare opportunity to regularly connect, one on one, with one of her children who had mysteriously grown into a fellow human being and had became a caregiver as well. So I satisfied myself with having the night off.

It turned out that I did get to go often enough that I became familiar with the regulars, and they with me. That familiarity led to another male member of the group asking a question specifically for me to answer. He and I were in similar situations as the primary caregiver for the woman we had been married to for most of our lives. He asked me how I reacted to seeing Judy so altered by the chemo that I didn't even recognize her. He said it had struck him one morning as he looked at his wife (who had never come to the group) while she sat at the table reading the paper. He was stunned by how much she had changed, at how he had to look carefully to see signs that it was even her.

I didn't know how to respond at first, mainly because I had not ever experienced what he was describing. So I changed his question a little and answered with something I had been reflecting on for a while and wanted to eventually say aloud sometime. The whole idea of viewing myself as a caregiver was strange to me. Caregiving itself was not, but identifying myself in that way was. I had started thinking about it when friends asked how I was holding up under the strain of Judy's illness. Those who asked wanted to make sure I was seeing to my own needs as well as Judy's. Like so much of the journey, especially the early part when things were happening so quickly, taking on the role of the caregiver and everything that implied was never specifically an issue I needed to consider. I just did everything out of immediate necessity. Until I was asked, I never gave it much thought, and to those who were asking, my response was something along the line of, "Oh, I'm doing all right," followed by something humorous enough to redirect the conversation.

But the queries regarding my own condition did get me thinking. At one point I even did some cleansing journal writing to address my concern that I wasn't more stressed by the circumstances than I was. Always ready to give myself a hard time, I interpreted the fact that I was taking it all in stride as an indication of how callous and unfeeling I was. After all, it was my Judy who was in such a dire way—Judy, the love of my life and my best friend for going on forty years. Writing about my feelings quickly got me past self-abuse and helped me reason out what really was going on with me. I even shared my thoughts with Judy as I worked through the dilemma. So when the group member asked me to explain myself, I was well prepared and ready to go public with my experience. It was the perfect opportunity.

"Oh, I don't know. Judy is still Judy to me. That never changes, even if she has. It's kind of like when people ask me how I'm holding up under all this. I don't see it as something I have to be holding up under. Rather it's something I have to do, something we have to do, and it comes automatically. When we signed up with our partners, when Judy and I decided to get married, we signed up for the long-term plan. And if we were going to be together that long, well, there was no way either of us was going to get through unscathed or unchanged. Something was going to happen. Something bad, something difficult, and probably a lot more than just once. These things, cancer, these kind of times—it's all part of the package. Happily-ever-after never meant not having difficulties.

"So this dealing with cancer, well, it's just a special time—one of those times that comes along every so often where we have to shift our focus a little, maybe a lot, and we have to step out of our usual roles and do something else that needs doing. It's not hard or difficult. I mean, it is, in the sense that it's scary and worrisome, and I often feel totally incompetent and more a hindrance than a help. But the other aspect to it, the bottom line part of it, is that we always knew we'd have to do it eventually. And, so in that regard, it's not hard on me, because under the circumstances, there's nothing else I'd rather be doing. It's a pleasure and a privilege to be doing this. It's what we wanted to be able to count on way back when. Now it's like it's all coming together just as we planned and hoped it would be. Even though nobody really plans for this, we all know it's going to come anyway."

I'm not sure that what I was trying to say ever became clear to the one who asked, or to the group. It probably sounded like bravado, the kind that comes when a person knows the worst is already past. Perhaps that played some part in my response. Still, even during the worst of Judy's bottoming out, I never felt overwhelmed, that fate had pushed me to the edge. I don't think there's anything special about the way I "held up" under it all. If nothing else, it was simple practicality. Becoming needy myself would have really created a mess, one I wouldn't have wanted, or trusted, anyone else to clean up. Besides, my falling apart in any way, shape, or form would have stolen Judy's thunder, and for the time being, at least, it was all about Judy.

That doesn't mean there wasn't a lot of heartache and anguish for me, along with all the satisfaction and even fun, during this time. It always gets back to the roller coaster. No one could ever stay high or low for very long. At one Qualife session, I was trying to infect a newcomer, also a caregiver, with a little hope and optimism, which she did not have when she arrived. As I spoke, I realized I was doing a terrible job, because for every positive memory I shared, I remembered and blurted out the low times that immediately followed. On and on I went, up and down and up and down, until the facilitator interrupted me to point out how much I wasn't helping. But others in the group jumped in to back me up, because the reality was just as I was describing. The ultimate lesson of caregiving and cancer was: don't let despair get you when you're down, and don't breathe too easily when you're up. Just be prepared to ride it out, because there's no getting off once the carny pulls the lever and the ride starts.

As the summer wore on, that "special time" was becoming more a thing of the past. Judy's weight was back, as was her exercise routine, as was her work. I no longer needed to take time off from my work. In the late spring, I had signed up for another writing workshop, feeling I then had the time and attention span to be able to write with the energy and enthusiasm it required. I submitted some chapters from the novel I had been working on for a couple of years and was encouraged enough by the feedback to commit myself to finishing a draft by the end of the summer and a rewrite by the end of the year. I finished the first draft while Judy was in Chicago visiting her sisters in September. I e-mailed her an announcement of that accomplishment, and she celebrated the news enthusiastically. Unspoken but understood between us was the more significant achievement of Judy finally feeling good enough to go on a trip that took her a thousand miles from her health care professionals.

Also that summer, in early August, our second grandson, Dominic, was born. Way back on the previous Christmas, when Darren told us that a grandchild was on the way, we couldn't muster up much enthusiasm. Our experiences back then with the miracle that is the human body had left us somewhat flat. We'd also had our fill of the miracles of modern medicine. But amazing events can occur in nine months. When Alma went into labor, Judy and I were right there at the hospital with her. The baby was in no hurry to be born, so Judy and I went home. We got the call after midnight that Dominic had arrived. Judy arose at dawn and returned to the hospital to see her brand new buddy.

We stayed with the support group at Qualife throughout the summer and fall. We no doubt would have stayed on longer had not financial matters forced Qualife to close its doors that December. At the final meeting of the support group, there was much talk of how continuing the group might be arranged. Everyone was reluctant to give it up, though no one ever articulated a practical plan for the future. In the course of that discussion, a student intern who had been assisting the facilitator pulled Judy and me aside. She told us we needn't feel obligated to stay with the group in whatever direction it was heading. She felt we were ready to move on, that Judy was ready to move on. At first that was an unsettling suggestion. But it only took a moment's reflection to see the value of it. It was time to stop defining our lives by Judy's cancer. It was time to move on.

12

Race for the Cure Reprise: The Gang's All Here

JUDY

We were riding high on being done with the difficult treatments, and we felt like celebrating. We talked about expanding our participation in Race for the Cure to the rest of the family. Then Dan got the excellent idea to expand it to friends. As one friend said, "Your house is a great location for a Race for the Cure party." We are just a few blocks from the start of the race course. I replied to her, "Did I have to get breast cancer just to be able to have a Race for the Cure party?" But the idea of inviting friends gave us the opportunity to say yet another thank-you for all the support we were receiving and to allow others to celebrate the recovery days with us.

October 2, 2004, was a beautiful Colorado day. I was decked in pink—T-shirt, hat, and feathered boa (a gift from Mary). I felt like a groupie, a part of the mob wearing colors, and I certainly was conscious of drawing attention to myself, not a comfortable thing for me. The thirty members of Team Judy marched with sixty-three thousand others. It was inspiring! It was the first Race for the Cure in which I walked with men (I had always participated in the women-only event in prior years), and that felt very good—men were certainly a big part of my life, and sharing this experience with them honored them and their support, while it gave them a chance to be part of the bigger picture of such a cause.

Two of our friends, Doug and Allison, made the Team Judy banner, and we had a lot of fun cheering for ourselves along the way, raising the banner up and showing it off to everyone. Another friend, Katherine, mentioned over and over how thrilling an event it was, how grand it was to be part of. She was seeing it through new eyes, and I could feel what she felt, even though I had been part of many Races for the Cure.

At the finish line, the announcer noticed our Team Judy banner and did her typical announcing and congratulating in welcoming us. I stopped at the announcer's tower to holler up to her and let her know that the Judy of Team Judy was me, Judy Gordon. The woman was someone I had worked with years earlier, and she choked up for a moment when she realized that of the masses she was welcoming, there were personal connections, too.

There was a gala celebration at the finish of the race, but by that time we had savored enough of the group effect and were eager to celebrate more intimately. So Team Judy marched through the crowd and back up to our house, where family and friends had the opportunity to be with one another.

That same day, Dan presented me with a very sweet letter commemorating our celebration. "We have had a full year of this epic episode, and on this day, we choose to celebrate life in your honor. Let me finally and formally get around to thanking you and appreciating you for all your efforts. This past year has not been about rescuing a damsel in distress. You have handled all this in a way that was right for you. You saw your needs and had them met. You understood that the immediate needs were important steps along the way to reaching the more distant goals. You reached out and called out and involved everyone you could. You were open and honest about the situation with everyone, choosing not to hide out and protect yourself, and at the same time choosing not to shield or protect others from the harsh realities of the disease. And it should come as no surprise that everyone is better for the experience."

Was I ever happy that we had reason to celebrate!

DAN

I don't remember exactly when we decided to have a party celebrating the year and Judy's survival of it. It may have been our idea or something someone else suggested. But walking in the Race for the Cure was naturally going to be a part of that celebration. Basically, we invited everyone to meet at our house, where we could enter the route several blocks after it started. Then we'd provide a brunch afterward for everyone who walked and for anyone who just wanted to drop by later. Darren, with two-month-old Dominic in tow, would man the house and direct latecomers while the rest of us walked.

As I have often done throughout our years together to commemorate a special event, I wrote Judy a letter, which I left for her to find when she woke that morning. (I can't help it—that's what I do.) In it, I tried to sift through a year's worth of emotions and events and thoughts to come up with the words that perfectly reflected what the year was all about. Considering how rapidly things changed, and how something critically important at a given moment quickly receded into old news, I doubt what I hoped to accomplish in that note was realistic. I have never reread what I wrote, but I do remember thanking her for insisting on doing things her way and then having the courage to be honest with everyone about what she was going through. We may have been throwing a party to thank and celebrate all who were part of our lives and our efforts that past year, but really it was just a big thank-you to Judy for what she gave us that year. And for still being around.

Thirty walkers gathered at our house that morning, and before the day was through at least that many more joined us at the house. Included among the walkers were Gail's husband, Doug, and their daughter Allison, who had made a sign for our group that read "TEAM JUDY," which we periodically held up to instigate some loud cheering. After practicing a time or two in front of the house, we made our way over to the course. We entered the route after the earlier, women-only event had gone by, but far enough ahead of the coed wave that for two-thirds of the route we had the street to ourselves. This allowed Judy and me to move among all who walked with us.

It was a far different experience for me from the previous year's event. I was there with Alex again, but also with quite a few more people. And instead of standing on the side as a spectator as thousands of women passed by, we were walking along the very same route. Thousands of women were way ahead of us, and thousands more—women, men, and children—were somewhere behind us, eager for their wave to be unleashed. And instead of me pontificating to Alex about cultural icons and bogeyman laureates, I was sharing moments of relief and gratefulness with assorted members of Team Judy. There was an irony to it all that I could only acknowledge and appreciate. It wasn't comeuppance; it was just irony, plain old benign, amazing irony. I don't regret where my mind had wandered that day the previous year while I observed the event. And I don't regret the past year's experiences that placed me out in the middle of the race a year later—especially since things turned out as they did. Judy and I have always enjoyed going for walks in the morning.

And it was a pleasant walk for the most part. There were several live music stations along the way and a fairly good-sized crowd of onlookers encouraging us on—since we were the only ones on the route at that time. About two-thirds of the way through the course, the coed wave of runners caught up with us. At first it was only the fastest and most serious runners—the ones trying to win the race.

Then it was the more recreational runners and then the joggers. The coed walkers obviously never caught up to us, but there were enough runners that we were soon surrounded, and Team Judy got dispersed in the crowd. It remained pretty chaotic from there to the finish line.

As we neared the finish line, we saw an old friend from Judy's earlier event-planning career. The woman was up on scaffolding with a microphone, urging the participants on and congratulating everyone as they crossed the finish line. When she saw our banner, she announced it to the crowd, "Here comes Team Judy; way to go, guys," unaware who the Judy was. Judy stopped at the finish line and called up to her. I was several feet back at the time and watched the announcer look down to see who was calling her name. She didn't recognize Judy at first, her hair only grown back to the length of a crew cut. Judy reintroduced herself, pointing to the pink shirt she wore to indicate she was a survivor. I watched the announcer put her hand to her mouth as it registered. Then, as Judy went on, the announcer turned away from the crowd for a moment to compose herself before rejoining the celebration.

Back at the house, the thirty people we had walked with quickly swelled by those who made the walk but never hooked up with the rest of Team Judy, and then swelled again when other friends dropped by as the morning and then the afternoon progressed. We had set things up so that people could eat and visit in comfort anywhere in the house and backyard, but for the most part everyone packed into the backyard, not wanting to splinter off, wanting to be part of a bigger whole. As impractical as that was, the backyard being pretty small, there was a sweetness to it that made the closeness more intimate than irritating. Everyone was in high spirits.

By midafternoon the celebration had thinned down to just family. Almost as if it had been scripted. And later, as evening approached, and after the various family members returned to their own homes and their own lives, Judy and I allowed ourselves a few quiet moments before she went upstairs to communicate with her sisters in Chicago about the day, and I went into the kitchen to clean up.

Staring out the kitchen window into the darkening, now empty yard, I wondered if something more planned should have been part of the day's celebration—like a few words from Judy or myself to the gathering, expressing our love and appreciation of them and our absolute joy at being able to share the day with our guests. That never happened, not in any formal way. But it couldn't have worked out better if it were planned. Instead, it happened in the exchanged words during embraces. It happened in the greetings as each person arrived, and in all the laughter and camaraderie that followed, and in our guests' parting words. Mostly those good-byes were hugs and muttered thanks, but there was also in them an unspoken understanding and sense that it was just good to be alive.

Epilogue

JUDY

When I was in the middle of chemo, I swore I would never say "yes" to such a regimen again. I did not think I would survive the treatment. But just two months after I completed chemo, I was able to say that I would choose treatment over no treatment if ever faced with that choice again. I don't typically spout "no pain, no gain" or "out of the darkness comes the light," but this powerful example may provide inspiration for future challenges.

The remainder of my treatment after our Race for the Cure celebration included six more months of weekly Herceptin infusions—and I thought less about them as treatments for myself and more about how my participation in the clinical trial was advancing the cause of treatments for all people with this kind of cancer. I was connected to a community, and I felt righteously noble.

The year 2005 was a year of feeling better, but I still felt somewhat fragile. After watching my body so long for side effects from treatment, it took a while for that "checking" instinct to fade away. Eventually my body seemed to settle down to an even keel. I was glad to have it back again.

During our time in the Qualife support group—February to December 2004—the group experienced no deaths. But within six months, two members died. Tom died in January, Bob in May. Then Margaret, in early 2006. Their deaths touched us deeply. We had gotten to know them, however briefly. We had all been on similar paths, but theirs had been shortened.

Cathlin's, too, was shortened. I didn't know Cathlin at the beginning of her cancer journey. She was initially diagnosed in the '80s. When I met her in 1998, she was producing a video on breast cancer survivors, and I was able to recommend another friend, Gina, to participate in that important project. When Cathlin's own cancer recurred several years later, it was a somber time. Yet she continued to live fully. I was awed by her ambitions, her physical and mental strength, and her self-awareness. When I was diagnosed, Cathlin was one of the first people I wanted to tell, and yet I didn't want to burden her. Her journey had been authentic and courageous in that she has always done what she wanted to do, to the level that she could control. I was so grateful that she was so candid with me about her experiences. I felt privileged that she included me in her confidences at the end of her life. She was always candid about what was happening to her and always interested to hear how I was doing. Having seen someone handle end-of-life so admirably and with authenticity made me less fearful.

Cathlin also helped me understand my mother's end-of-life better. She didn't do so intentionally, but her experience provided an insight. My mother had been stoic; she didn't talk about her cancer experience, and when she heard that it was terminal, she was ready to die. The quality of life she had been used to was the only one she could envision, and if it was not to be, she didn't want to live any longer. Cathlin, on the other hand, kept redefining the issue of quality of life as the cancer reduced her abilities and her options. I appreciated seeing that adaptability—there is not one right way, but there are many ways, and more is possible at the end of life than most of us can imagine.

Cathlin died on October 5, 2004—just two days after our Race for the Cure celebration.

My friend Gina was first diagnosed in 1998, at the same time that both of our mothers were dying of cancer. Gina is ten years younger than me. I felt privileged to be present at her treatments, to witness someone wanting to survive. And she did so in strong fashion—she was a role model of strength. It surprised me that when I told her of my diagnosis, she admitted that her strength felt shaken. It was as if she had not truly experienced the emotional impact of her own cancer until she heard about mine. Although Gina's breast cancer recurred in 2005, as of this writing it is in remission.

DAN

A couple of weeks after the race-day celebration, Judy and I took a vacation. We drove down to Sedona, Arizona for a few days, staying at a bed and breakfast. We had never been there before, but were intrigued by its location, its natural beauty, and its vortexes of spiritual energy. It was a relaxing escape. We hiked a lot, ate well, soaked in a hot tub, and when Judy was napping or going to sleep early, I worked on my novel. On our last day there Judy persuaded me to submit to my first massage—by which I mean the first one that I had to pay for. It was a pleasant enough experience, though not one I have repeated since.

Afterward, I turned the tables and told Judy that since we were experiencing firsts, I thought she should have a psychic reading. My experience with psychics was not vast, but I had recently had a couple of readings, partly from curiosity and partly because my novel had a psychic character, and I felt I should know a little about psychics and their process. I found my readings to be positive, affirming experiences, which made me wonder what a down-to-earth, practical person like Judy would have to say about it. She came out of the reading upbeat but not yet ready to talk about it.

On the road the next day, driving through the sparse and stark landscape of the Navajo reservation in northern Arizona, we listened to the tape of Judy's reading. Unfortunately, it was a poor recording, and with the interference of the car noise, we could not clearly hear what was being said. So Judy told me about it. She began by commenting how accurately the reader had picked up and presented details about her. She, too, found the process somewhat fascinating and certainly positive. It probably wouldn't be good for the industry, we decided, if the readers spouted out doom and gloom. By accentuating the positive, there was a stronger likelihood of return business. Rays of hope never hurt anyone, and even helped, if they got people thinking that good things could happen, and maybe even spurred them to take the steps to make good things happen.

Judy then explained how the reader used Tarot cards and how some of the key cards spoke to who she was and how she did things. She felt that the cards accurately pegged her. Then she said the reader also looked at her palm. The reader saw a break in the lifeline, at a place about four-fifths of the total length. When Judy revealed her recent ordeal with cancer, the reader agreed that might be what the break indicated. Doing the math on that, Judy being fifty-six, and that representing 80 percent of the whole, indicated that Judy's palm had her life span at seventy years. She told me that without emotion, simply relating to me what had been discussed at the reading.

I suppose it was a good thing that she was driving at the time and not me, because that little tidbit stunned me, like nothing in the year since the diagnosis had. It took me a few minutes to digest, and then a few minutes more to formulate how I was going to ask what I had to ask next.

"So, Judy," I began uncertainly. "Seventy years. You seem to be taking that rather calmly. I wouldn't have expected that from you. Only seventy years? What's with that? Did you just dismiss it as the wild guess of some charlatan psycho-psychic who really has no way of knowing, so it's not worth getting worked up about?"

"Oh, no," she said. "I don't know if there is any reason to believe that reader over anybody else, but it matches what I wanted to believe. So there's no reason to be upset. I'm kind of relieved. It confirms what I was hoping for."

That really did me in. That was not the Judy I knew and thought I had back. That was not the someone who was tickled by life—*that* Judy would have kept saying "do that again," not "seventy will be plenty."

"OK. Slow down," I said. "I seem to be missing some critical information here. I am the one who doesn't want to live long. You are the one who wants to keep going and going. Has something changed here? You *are* my first wife, aren't you?"

Then she told me that at one point during the worst of the chemo treatments, when she was sure something had gone wrong and she was dying, she put it out to the Universe that she would like to live until she was seventy. Surviving the chemo, she took as a good sign. Having her wish confirmed the day before by a randomly selected, impartial, totally objective source was validating. She was still happy with the arrangement she had made and was content to accept just those remaining years and make the most of them.

Maybe she was, but I wasn't. I had to act quickly to counteract the deal she had made, before it became a self-fulfilling prophecy. Seventy was only fourteen years away. "Only fourteen. Just think of how fast the last fourteen years have gone. Fourteen is a very finite number—ten fingers and four toes. It's not way out in the future. It's just, well, around the next corner. That's hardly enough time to have new careers, new homes, and several major changes in our lives. We may very well be on the last lap."

When the frantic panic approach didn't seem to get to her, I tried tugging at some more sensitive strings. "In fourteen years, Spencer won't even have his driver's license. He'll be in high school. An adolescent. It'll be a hard enough time for him already. And Dominic won't even be in high school yet. He'll still be a kid. And Maria will hopefully be in college. Or maybe thinking about getting married. You want to miss her wedding?"

But Judy was unmoved. Without putting it into words, she was letting me know that things had changed. Her undeniable fears regarding cancer and its consequences were no longer major players in her life. Her love of life hadn't changed. If anything, it had intensified. And if you live life that way, any number of years is enough, because any number of years—no matter how many—would be too few.

Anyway, I was probably getting all worked up for nothing, and what really bothered me was the thought of being around after she was gone. I had been so sure for so long that I would go first and she'd have to deal with losing me that I suddenly felt very fragile and unprepared for the other possibility. Even if I understood that it ain't necessarily going to play out that way, the number fourteen seems way too little for all the life we still have in front of us. And, now, at this writing, it's already down to eleven.

So I guess that despite whatever spin anyone chooses to put on their cancer experience, the bottom line is that it is all about death. That makes it the experience it is. Once the diagnosis is made, all that's left are victims and survivors. And the only way to avoid being a victim is to be a survivor long enough to die of something else. Again, it is a quirk of our culture that cancer has become such a big-time player. Perhaps our culture's reluctance to accept death has made cancer so big. What causes cancer and what prevents cancer have been hot topics for the last fifty years, as if by avoiding what causes it and embracing what prevents it we believe that we can cheat death.

As I've already said, I don't expect that immortality thing to become a reality anytime soon. That kind of leaves us with the ageless debate concerning quantity versus quality. That's what Judy encountered and resolved on her journey. If a close encounter with cancer does nothing else, its threat to quantity will focus attention on quality. It's as if some master plan is at work to make us reassess what we value and what is valuable—and that plan is coming together beautifully.

Surely this must have happened for a reason.

JUDY

My last journal entry, October 22, 2004: *So I look in the mirror, and I look like myself again—I have put on all the weight I lost last year (It would have been nice to have kept some of it off!). My activities are back to normal—I am even doing yoga at least once every other week. My conversations with others don't include the worried looks or serious "how are you's."* I'm glad to move on.

I'm more glad to be able to move on basically intact.

And I'm most glad that I was able to do the cancer journey in a way that let me be me. I know that previous generations were more likely to keep personal challenges to themselves. There were taboos, formally or informally, about sharing bad news with others. That doesn't work for many of us today. We are more verbal, we see more options, and the vast and continual changes in our lives have forced us to develop more flexible and open ways in dealing with issues. My mother and father responded to their cancers in ways that were typical of their upbringing. But I felt sadness for both of them (and for myself) that their experiences didn't allow more personal interaction and conversation, didn't offer more enlightenment to those of us close to them. Trying to handle something as big as cancer on your own has to be a very lonely and difficult thing. I, on the other hand, have let it flow through me and out of me in journal writing, in conversations, in correspondence, and in visible emotions, and I feel healed in numerous ways. The number of my days is not guaranteed, but I see them differently now. And I believe I have modeled for others an openness and authenticity that may be of help along any unwelcome journey they travel. I'm glad to have uncovered a way that worked for me.

Mary's son Nick, long a friend of ours in his own right, wrote this to me during the course of my treatments: "Sometimes we need to see other people do something that's scary first, and then we can start to step into the unknown ourselves. So many times we are asked to 'let go' in order to grow, but can't because we're afraid. Watching someone else do it first is sometimes all we need in order to take those first steps ourselves. Your experience of journeying into the unknown and surrendering to forces out of your control, the 'you' you always took yourself to be, is a miracle and something to be shared."

I hope this tale will be of value to those who may experience such an unwelcome journey in the future.

About the Authors

Judy is a writer by profession. She writes how-to publications for nonprofit clients. In 1999, Judy authored *Parenting Our Daughters: For Parents and Other Caring Adults*, published by Girls Count, a Denver-based organization. She is a member of the Colorado Authors League.

Dan is a writer by avocation. He has written personal essays and opinion columns, but most of his work has been fiction. He uses his writing to explore and hopefully gain insight into the human condition. Dan has a thirty-year career in retail.

The authors have been married to each other since 1970. They were high school sweethearts who wed upon college graduation. They and their two adult sons and their growing families live in Denver, Colorado.

When Judy was diagnosed with breast cancer in 2003 at age fifty-five, Judy and Dan shared the cancer journey together. And they shared the writing of this memoir.

www.theheroicsoffallingapart.com

www.ingramcontent.com/pod-product-compliance
Lightning Source LLC
Chambersburg PA
CBHW051412280526
45785CB00003B/1038